Trends in Oral Health Care

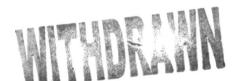

Also available by the same editor from Quay Books, MA Healthcare Ltd:

Trends in Wound Care, volume I

Trends in Wound Care, volume II

Trends in Oral Health Care
BJN monograph

edited by
Richard White

Quay Books
MA Healthcare Limited

Quay Books Division, Mark Allen Publishing Limited, Jesses Farm,
Snow Hill, Dinton, Wiltshire, SP3 5HN

British Library Cataloguing-in-Publication Data
A catalogue record is available for this book

© Mark Allen Publishing Ltd 2004
ISBN 1 85642 226 7

Printed in the UK by Cromwell Press, Trowbridge

Contents

List of contributors

Jane Ball is Staff Nurse, Surgery, The Newark Hospital, Newark.

Pauline Chilton is Staff Nurse, Medicine, The Newark Hospital, Newark.

Joan Curzio, Professor of Practice Development, South Bank University, Faculty of Health, Harold Wood Hospital, Essex.

Karen Gill is Staff Nurse, Surgery, The Newark Hospital, Newark.

Amanda Honnor is Macmillan Nurse, Palliative Care Team, University Hospital of Leicester.

Christine V Jones was formerly Senior Tutor Dental Hygienist, School of Dental Hygiene, Birmingham Dental Hospital.

Annie Law is Practitioner/Lecturer, Directorate of Cancer Services and Clinical Haematology, University Hospitals of Leicester.

Louise Lee is Macmillan Clinical Nurse Specialist, The Newark Hospital, Newark.

Maggie McCowan is Senior Nurse Infection Control, National Waiting Times Centre, Clydebank, Glasgow.

Karen McEwan is Ward Manager, Medicine, The Newark Hospital, Newark.

Lin Perry is Senior Researcher, Faculty of Health and Social Care Sciences, Kingston University/St George's Hospital Medical School, Kingston-upon-Thames, Surrey.

Penny Pickering is Staff Nurse, Medicine, The Newark Hospital, Newark.

Josephine Roberts is Ward Sister, Lord Byron Ward, Brookfields Hospital, Cambridge.

Lynn Smart is Ward Manager, Surgery, The Newark Hospital, Newark.

Dr Jean Watkins was a partner at the Alma Partnership, The Winton Health Centre, Bournemouth.

Richard White is a freelance Medical Writer and Clinical Research Consultant, Whitstone, Cornwall.

Val White is Macmillan Clinical Nurse Specialist, The Newark Hospital, Newark.

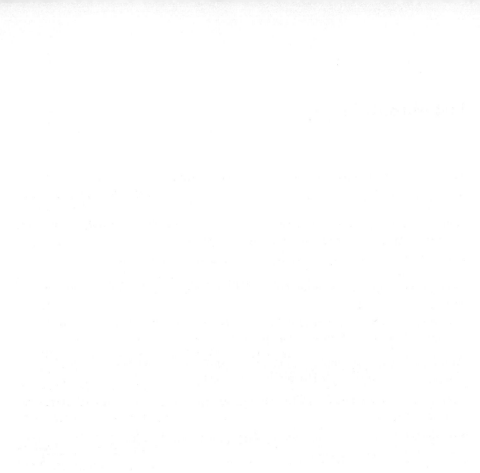

Foreword

In my early career I wrote that, 'it is often the simplest procedures that are most in need of scrutiny, for these are the aspects of nursing practice which are taken for granted and have become firmly incorporated into the routinised fabric of nursing'. Oral assessment and care of the mouth is a superb example of one such 'simple' procedure. Twenty years on, oral care has still not received the research scrutiny it deserves, nor is sufficient education and emphasis given to ensure that interventions are effective. Oral care is often delivered in a ritualised manner, without reference to a patient's individual needs or the evidence base for practice. Most oral care is delegated to junior nurses in spite of the fact that it requires skill and expertise. There is a real danger that oral care can become a Cinderella activity when workload is high and staffing levels are low.

This collection of related chapters is derived from articles recently published in the *British Journal of Nursing*. It presents an overall picture of the current knowledge base in oral care and raises awareness of oral health and dysphagia. Its focus on recommended standards of practice in different clinical settings provides a unique and up-to-date resource and this is enhanced by the glossary with photographs which aid identification of common mouth conditions.

The message from this book is clear. Much more education in oral health procedures is required for nurses and all other healthcare practitioners. Oral health must be promoted as a key element in the everyday practice of nursing for all patient groups. This book provides a background from which both students and practising nurses can develop their knowledge and skills in this area and take pride in providing the highest quality of oral care.

Professor Dame Jill Macleod Clark
Southampton
September 2003

Introduction

The oral health status of the general patient population — whether in hospital or in the community — is all too frequently overlooked. This is a mistake as the mouth can be a useful pointer to disease states and nutritional status, as well as being of great impact on patient quality of life. This collection of related chapters focuses on aspects of oral health, its assessment and treatment in different clinical settings. A detailed glossary covers the common terms of oral disease conditions with photographs to illustrate typical presentations and a basic assessment procedure. It is hoped that this book will provide a useful introduction and reference aide to student and practising nurses, medical and dental students, and carers in general.

Richard White
Whitstone, Cornwall
July 2003

1

Oral health assessment: a review of current practice

Richard White

Introduction

The assessment of oral health status and related care of patients is a largely neglected area of nursing and general medical practice unless the patient presents with a specific oral problem (White, 2000). With the notable exceptions of high-risk patient groups, such as those receiving chemotherapy, in neonatal and intensive care units, and in terminal care, few patients enjoy regular, formal oral assessments and care (Lee *et al*, 2001). Interventions such as nurse administered oral hygiene, should not be reserved only for high-risk groups but ideally be provided to all patients, whether in hospital or in the community, as they can reveal signs and symptoms of oral disease, manifestations of systemic disease, drug side-effects, or trauma; and, provide important diagnostic clues (Jones, 1998; Roberts, 2000a, b, c: see *Chapter 2*).

This chapter sets out to review the *status quo* in oral healthcare as described in the published literature; also, to emphasise further the need for nurse and carer education and provide a literature review and introduction to common oral health problems. It also sets out to establish the rationale for oral assessment in all contexts of patient care. It is not an objective to provide yet another assessment tool, but instead to emphasise the need for a strategy and use of existing tools. The criteria for identification of an appropriate tool have been outlined by Roberts (2000c, and in *Chapter 2*).

Disease or trauma to the mouth can exacerbate the patients' general medical condition and reduce their quality of life. As will be shown, disease may result in reduced or inability to eat or swallow, further compromising health. Poor oral hygiene has also been shown to predispose the elderly, infirm patient to chest infections and coronary heart disease (Loesche *et al*, 1998).

Oral hygiene should be a significant feature of nursing care. Crosby (1989) states that, 'care of the mouth is considered to be one of the most basic of nursing activities'. However, the available literature reveals a different picture; the nurse's knowledge of oral health problems is often limited (Longhurst, 1998). This is frequently due to the absence of oral health education at the pre-qualification stage (Boyle, 1992). In clinical practice, oral health is often not regarded as a priority (Shepherd *et al*, 1987) even though there are standard texts that include examination of the mouth and throat (Scully, 2000; Johnson, 2002). There may be no local 'enthusiasm' or culture reflected by the absence of assessment tools or protocols for oral health. Consequently, on admission to hospital or presentation in the community, the patient is usually asked questions related to dentures and not thoroughly assessed. An excellent opportunity to address any oral health problems is therefore missed. While oral health assessment should be a feature of the care of all patients in both community and hospital, there are key areas where circumstances dictate special attention be given to the mouth. The main 'at risk' patient groups are listed in *Table 1.1*.

Table 1.1: Patient groups 'at risk' for oral health

Patients receiving:	intensive care, chemotherapy, oxygen therapy, immunosuppressive therapy, ie. transplant patients
Patients with cancer	
Patients receiving palliative care	
The elderly	
Neonates, especially pre-term	
Diabetics	
Patients who are nutritionally compromised	

In the intensive care unit (ITU) patients are often unconscious and may be mechanically ventilated or receiving continuous nasal oxygen; these all predispose to oral problems, although, if the patient is hydrated adequately with intravenous fluids the mouth should not dry out. In a review of oral care in the ITU, Fitch *et al* (1999) found that in the USA few nurses were formally trained in assessing, and oral care protocols were rare. They also found that by training nurses in assessment and implementing oral care protocols, the oral health of patients in the ITU could be improved.

Patients receiving radiotherapy, chemotherapy or high doses of anti-neoplastic drugs are well known to be at very high risk of oral health problems, indeed age, immunosuppression and renal disease further increase risk (Richardson, 1987; Berger and Eilers, 1998). Patients with cancer are especially vulnerable to oral problems (Crosby, 1989; Lee *et al*, 2001) and need high standards of oral assessment and care; they may be receiving chemotherapy with cytotoxic drugs, which are well known to provoke ulceration, xerostomia, and secondary infection of the oral cavity (Richardson, 1987; see *Chapter 5* and the *Glossary* for common terminology and *Table 1.2* for drugs with oral manifestations). Radiotherapy is also associated with oral problems such as pain, xerostomia, reduced saliva and dysphagia (see *Chapter 7*), particularly when directed at head and neck tumours. Myelosuppression (eg. with busulphan or hydroxyurea) or immunosuppression results in neutropenia and thrombocytopenia, thereby increasing the risks of infection, particularly candidiasis in the mouth. The importance of oral care for the cancer patient has been emphasised by Allbright (1984):

> *Oral complications cause the patient much misery and discomfort and may contribute to more serious complications such as systemic infections and nutritional impairment, both causes of morbidity in cancer patients.*

Table 1.2: Oral side-effects of some commonly used drugs

Drug	Side-effect
Diuretics	Glossodynia
Anticholinergics, eg. hyoscine, some anti-emetics	Dry mouth
Antimuscarinics for parkinsonism	Dry mouth
Antibiotics	Candidiasis, hairy tongue, Stevens-Johnson syndrome
Opioid analgesics, eg. diconal	Dry mouth
Tricyclics, eg. amitryptiline	Dry mouth
MAOI antidepressives	Dry mouth
Metronidazole	Altered taste
Penicillamine	Altered taste
Phenytoin	Swelling (hypertrophy) of the gingivae
Methotrexate	Stomatitis
Retinoids	Dry mouth, erosions

The elderly, whether at home, in hospital, or in residential accommodation are also a high-risk group (Roberts, 2000a; *Chapter 2*). The clinical picture is often confused by chronic illnesses which have oral manifestations such as diabetes (both insulin-dependent and non-insulin dependent), rheumatoid disease (note that reduced manual dexterity may impair teeth/denture cleaning), inadequate diet, and frequently, poorly fitting dentures (see *Table 1.3* for oral manifestations of systemic disease). Do not assume that if the patient is alert they have no oral health problems and are conducting oral hygiene themselves. Initial and regular ongoing assessment is necessary (Hallett, 1984; Roberts, 2000b, c and *Chapter 2*).

Table 1.3: Oral manifestations of systemic disease

Disease	Characteristic
Diabetes	Candidiasis, glossodynia, ketone breath and xerostomia in diabetic ketoacidosis
Acquired immune deficiency syndrome	Candidiasis, erosive gingivitis, aphthous ulceration, Kaposi's sarcoma
Pemphigus	Tense blisters which rupture to leave non-healing ulcers
Rheumatoid (Sjogren's syndrome)	Dry mouth
Acute leukaemia	Gingival hypertrophy (gross)
Bronchiectasis/RTI	Halitosis (foul breath)
Malignancy	Stomatitis. Leukoplakia or ulcer on the tongue. Chronic ulceration of the lip
Lichen planus	Lace-like pattern of white lines on buccal mucosae
Stevens-Johnson syndrome	Blistering and erosions of the lips
Macroglossia	Myxoedema, amyloidosis, tumour
Scurvy	Swollen gums with bleeding

Mouth problems in the terminally ill can cause great distress and seriously reduce quality of life. Denton (1999) has shown that in this patient group mouth care can be an indicator of the level of nursing care that the patient receives. These patients, regardless of their state of debility, may benefit from oral care (Lee, 2001 and *Chapter 4*). Typically, problems such as xerostomia, candidiasis (Pople and Oliver, 1986), gingivitis and ulceration, and, herpes simplex are encountered. The underlying disease may give rise to mouth problems, eg. leukaemia, as may the treatments, eg. radiotherapy, cytotoxics, steroids, antibiotics; or, the problem may be exacerbated by dehydration through poor fluid intake, mouth breathing, or oxygen therapy. Halitosis may not distress the patient but may cause embarrassment and concern relatives, the cause should be investigated and corrective measures taken. Turner (1994) has published a comprehensive guide on assessment and care for this group of patients.

Premature infants, and children with developmental difficulties, special needs, lactose intolerance, gastric reflux (Boyd *et al*, 1998), and cerebral palsy (Pope and Curzon, 1991) are all at risk for oral health problems. Furthermore, their inability to communicate verbally requires that they be examined regularly.

Immunosuppression will often give rise to oral problems. Whether by drug therapy or through disease, suppression of the immune response will allow opportunistic infections such as candidiasis to develop. Patients with human immunodeficiency virus (HIV) disease have been shown to suffer widely from oral problems. In a recent study, Coates *et al* (1996) showed 32% of a sample of HIV patients to have oral candida infection, 24% to have leukoplakia, 33% periodontitis and 18% gingivitis. As with any other patient group, mouth disease on this scale is likely to impair nutritional intake and so further compromise the health of the subject.

The relationship between oral care and nutrition has been clearly established (Watson, 1989; Jones, 1998 and *Chapter 6*). According to Jones, 'scant attention has been paid to the specific relationship between oral care and nutrition intake' and Watson (1989) claims that nutritional intake is impaired by lack of attention to oral care — or lack of knowledge of the patient's oral state. As well as reduced or poor nutritional intake, dysphagia may be a factor in malnutrition and dehydration (Perry, 2001 and *Chapter 7*).

The list of risk factors in *Table 1.5* illustrates clearly the wide range of patients that are 'at risk' and should, therefore, be assessed.

The state of health in the mouth will have an important influence on the patients' general health. Maintenance of good oral

Table 1.5: Risk factors for reduced oral feeding

Debility
Anorexia
Nausea
Vomiting
Dysphagia
Local tumour
Weakness
Mouth odour
Anticholinergic drugs
Local irradiation
Malignant ulceration
Chemotherapy
Dehydration

Source: Jones, 1998

hygiene can preclude the development of more serious illness. For example, several studies have established a link between oral (dental) disease and heart disease (Loesche *et al*, 1998). In a study on US veterans, the authors confirmed a link between coronary heart disease and oral health parameters, such as xerostomia and pathogen colonisation of the mouth. The implication being that attention to oral hygiene will reduce heart disease. It has been postulated (Limeback, 1998) that infections such as pneumonia are also caused by oral pathogenic micro-organisms. In the institutionalised care of the elderly, Limeback believes that aspiration of fluids from the oropharynx introduce pathogens to the lower respiratory tract. These pathogens, known to colonise dental plaque, have flourished in the mouth due to poor hygiene. This theory is supported by the finding that in patients undergoing open heart surgery, pre-rinsing the mouth with the antibacterial chlorhexidine gluconate significantly lowered the mortality rate from post-surgical pneumonia (De Riso and Ladowski, 1996).

Assessment

The conduct of oral health assessment should be defined in a protocol which defines the procedure, frequency and follow-up (including referral procedures, *Figure 1.1*). The practicalities of using a single protocol for varying and very different areas of medicine or nursing outweigh the need for multiple protocols. The important step is to implement a formal assessment protocol. Turner (1996) has defined the role of the nurse in the provision of oral care and has outlined the basic principles of assessment. The key features of assessment and of signs and symptoms of oral disease have been widely published (Schweigner, 1980; Roberts, 1986; Richardson, 1987; Field, 1998).

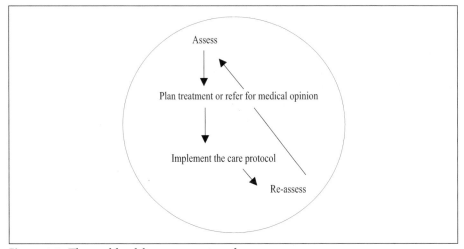

Figure 1.1: The oral health assessment cycle

Numerous authors have addressed the issues: Maurer (1977) suggested that an oral assessment be conducted on admission and included in the general admission procedure, and that adequate provision should be made in the nursing process for the conduct and recording of this assessment. Little progress appears to have been made in this area since.

Boyle (1992) has proposed a strategy for mouth care, a key precursor to the implementation of protocols and assessments. In this important 'health promotion' strategy there are five elements:

- oral assessment criteria and standards that can be used by all grades of nursing staff
- a continuing education programme for all grades of staff
- a ward based programme
- a multidisciplinary team approach to mouth care (involving nursing, dental, occupational therapy staff, and dieticians)
- improved referral and feedback mechanisms.

Education should involve experienced staff, particularly those with relevant backgrounds, eg. dental hygienists. When assessing, take care to be gentle and do not increase the patient's anxiety through rough manipulation of the tongue and cheeks. A gentle approach will help in future assessments of the patient.

In the USA, Miller and Rubenstein (1987) showed newly qualified nurses to be untrained in assessments of patients' oral health requirements. In the UK nurses are inadequately trained in oral health assessment and care. Little or no priority is given to this essential aspect of care. As recently as 1998, Longhurst has highlighted the deficiencies in nurse education in oral health. In a survey of all 162 nurse training establishments, many had syllabus deficiencies. For example, of the respondents providing pre-registration teaching, 79% had no dental input, only 28% taught the use of an oral assessment form, and 38% had no exclusive lectures on oral care. In addition, students were often recommended books that had insufficient information to provide an insight into oral care or mouth disease. Longhurst lists key textbooks and journal articles that fulfil such needs. Specific guides to oral health and disease for nurses can supplement this list (Roberts, 1986; Field, 1998); in addition, there are informative textbooks on oral medicine with excellent colour plates (Tyldesley, 1988; Toghill, 1990).

The situation with regards to the education of qualified nurses is equally neglected. Adams (1996) has reviewed the literature and surveyed nursing staff with respect to knowledge of oral health matters. She found that:

In my clinical experience, as a ward sister on an acute medical ward for elderly patients, oral care is generally a neglected area of nursing in terms of assessment and actual care given. If this is indeed the case, then many nurses are guilty of misconduct according to the UKCC.

It has been over twenty years since Macleod-Clarke and Hockey (1979) stated that:

It is often the simplest procedures that are most in need of scrutiny, for these are the aspects of nursing practice which are taken for granted and have become firmly incorporated into the routinised fabric of nursing.

More recently it has been established (Crosby, 1989) that a patient's oral health status is a good indicator of the care given; implying that poor status is attributable to inadequate care. A brief survey by Hatton-Smith (1994) found that oral care was given in a ritualised manner, without reference to a patient's individual needs. Most oral care is delegated to junior nurses and is described by nurses as an unpleasant task (Boyle, 1992). Reduced staffing levels affect oral care and, accordingly, this is given less priority than more obvious areas (Speedie, 1983).

Assessment tools

In the last twenty-five years there have been many publications offering oral assessment tools and guidelines for their use. No single tool appears to have achieved pre-eminence; however, this need not cause confusion. The single most important step forward in patient oral health is to acknowledge the need for assessment, then select a tool from the following list. The selection can be based on the needs of a specific patient group, otherwise select a general tool using the criteria for selection defined by Roberts (2000c, *Chapter 2*). De Walt's oral guide (1975) identified nine key areas for assessment (see below) but gave no guidelines to risk assessment. Maurer (1977) built on the De Walt tool but without addressing risk (*Table 1.6*).

Table 1.6: Key areas and features to assess (after De Walt, 1975)
Saliva: note too much as well as too little
Tongue moisture: relate to different regions
Tongue colour and texture
Palate moisture
Gingival tissues
Colour of membranes
Lip texture: note presence of any lesions, note cheilitis
Lip moisture: note dryness and fissuring
Soft tooth debris

Richardson (1987) and Heals (1993) have provided quite detailed assessment tools and rationale for cancer patients. Schweiger *et al* (1980) devised a detailed assessment that gathered diagnostic information on the patient's general health. Eilers *et al*'s Oral Assessment Guide (1988) includes advice on frequency of assessment. Frequency of assessment is the nurses' responsibility and depends entirely on the patient's needs. Jenkins' oral 'at risk' calculator (1989) was designed for the ITU; it gives a risk 'weighting' to different factors and emphasises the need to tailor care and frequency to the needs of each individual patient. Atchinson and Dolan (1990) have devised a general oral health assessment index for the elderly. Both Jenkins (1989) and Heals (1993) have devised tools very similar in appearance and use to the Norton Pressure Sore Score (1962) and are, therefore, likely to be recognised and familiar to many nurses. Jones (1998), in an article on oral hygiene and nutrition, outlines aims and objectives for mouth care and offers a simple assessment tool.

Formal measures for assessing oral health include the Western Consortium for Cancer Nursing Research (WCCNR) staging system, the Oral Assessment Guide (OAG), and the World Health Organization Mucositis Grading System (Anon, 1991).

The tool is only as good as the basic understanding that the nurse has of oral health. The nurse must be able to recognise key features of oral disease and trauma and to know when to refer the patient for medical opinion. The *Glossary* defines the common terminology of oral disease conditions together with representative photographs of some disease conditions.

Oral health should be a central part of nursing and medical care. There are numerous, recent publications drawing attention to disturbing deficiencies in education and care giving. This requires urgent rectification. To achieve this, all nurses, junior doctors and carers need education — not only as students, but while in post as practising nurses. The adoption of a strategy, such as that advocated by Boyle, would be a significant step forward in improving patient oral health. The good oral health of patients is achieved through the co-operation and collaboration of informed carers in providing adequate nutrition, oral hygiene, fully functioning healthy teeth or dentures and, normal salivation and swallowing. The presence of disease in the mouth or trauma to the mouth will compromise this. The well-trained, observant nurse should have access to and training in the use of a validated assessment tool for oral health status, and time to follow a defined protocol for the administration of mouth care for the patient. To achieve this, oral hygiene must be acknowledged as a clinical priority. Oral assessment should be conducted on a patient's admission and at appropriate intervals thereafter, according to clinical need; it should also be included and recorded in the general admission procedures.

Key points

⌘ Oral health and hygiene are important for patient quality of life and general health.

⌘ Adopt a strategy for assessment and care.

⌘ All patients/clients should have an oral health assessment on admission and at regular intervals. Document assessments.

⌘ Identify 'at risk' patients and assess accordingly.

⌘ Plan oral care.

⌘ Nurses should be trained in oral health assessment and mouth care.

⌘ Neglecting patient oral health care is a breach of the UKCC's *Code of professional conduct* (1992). It increases patient morbidity, mortality, and costs to the healthcare system.

References

Adams R (1996) Qualified nurses lack of adequate knowledge related to oral health, resulting in inadequate oral care of patients on medical wards. *J Adv Nurs* **24**(3):552–60

Allbright A (1984) Oral care for the cancer chemotherapy patient. *Nurs Times* **80**(21): 40–2

Anon (1991) Development of a staging system for chemotherapy — induced stomatitis. Western Consortium for Cancer Research Nursing. *Cancer Nurse* **14**: 1, 6–12

Atchison KA, Dolan TA (1990) Development of the Geriatric Oral Health Assessment Index. *J Dent Educ* **54**(11): 680–7

Berger AM, Eilers J (1998) Factors influencing oral cavity status during high-dose antineoplastic therapy: a secondary data analysis. *Oncol Nurs Forum* **25**(9): 1623–6

Boyd LD, Palmer C, Dwyer JT (1998) Managing oral health related nutrition issues of high-risk infants and children. *J Clin Pediatr Dent* **23**(1): 31–6

Boyle S (1992) Assessing mouth care. *Nurs Times* **88**(15): 44–6

Coates E, Slade GD, Goss AN, Gorkic E (1996) Oral conditions and their social impact among HIV dental patients. *Aust Dent J* **4**(1): 33–6

Crosby C (1989) Method in mouth care. *Nurs Times* **85**(35): 38–41

De Riso AJ, Ladowski JS (1996) Chlorhexidine gluconate oral rinse reduces respiratory infection in patients undergoing heart surgery. *Chest* **109**(6): 1556–61

De Walt E (1975) Effect of timed hygiene measures on oral mucosa in a group of elderly subjects. *Nurse Res* **24**(1): 22–7

Denton E (1999) Mouthcare — an indicator of the level of nursing care a patient receives? *J Community Nursing* **13**(11): 8–11

Eilers J, Berger A, Petersen M (1988) Development, testing and application of the oral assessment guide. *Oncol Nurs Forum* **15**(3): 325–30

Field D (1998) Mouth care-1. *Nurs Times* **94**(7): suppl 1–2; Practical procedures for nurses — 9.2. Mouth care-2. *Nurs Times* **94**(8): suppl 1–2

Fitch JA, Munro CL, Glass CA, Pellegrini JM (1999) Oral care in the adult intensive care unit. *Am J Crit Care* **8**(5): 314–8

Hallett N (1984) Mouthcare. *Nurs Mirror* **159**(21): 31–3

Hatton-Smith CK (1994) A last bastion of ritualised practice? A review of nurses' knowledge of oral healthcare. *Prof Nurse* **9**(5): 304–8

Heals D (1993) A key to wellbeing. Oral hygiene in patients with advanced cancer. *Prof Nurse* **8**(6): 391–8

Jenkins DA (1989) Oral care in the ICU: an important nursing role. *Nurs Standard* **8**(4): 24–8

Johnson W (2002) Head and neck. In: Cross S, Rimer M, eds. *Nurse Practitioner Manual of Clinical Skills.* Baillière Tindall, RCN Publications London

Jones CV (1998) The importance of oral hygiene in nutritional support. *Br J Nurs* **7**(2): 74–83

Lee L, White V, Ball K *et al* (2001) An audit of oral care practice and staff knowledge in hospital palliative care. *Int J Palliative Nurs* **7**(8): 395–400

Limeback H (1998) Implications of oral infections on systemic diseases in the institutionalised elderly with a special focus on pneumonia. *Ann Periodontol* **3**(1): 262–75

Loesche WJ *et al* (1998) Assessing the relationship between dental disease and coronary heart disease in elderly US veterans. *J Am Dent Assoc* **129**(3): 301–11

Longhurst RH (1998) A cross-sectional study of the oral healthcare instruction given to nurses during their basic training. *Br Dent J* **184**(9): 453–7

Macleod-Clarke J, Hockey L (1979) *Research for Nursing.* HM&M Publications, Aylesbury

Maurer J (1977) Providing optimal oral health. *Nurs Clin North America* **12**(4): 67–85

Miller R, Rubenstein L (1987) Oral care for hospital patients. *J Nurs Educ* **26**(9): 362–7

Norton D, Maclaren R, Exton-Smith AN (1962) *An Investigation of Geriatric Nursing Problems in Hospital: National corporation for the care of old people.* Churchill Livingstone, Edinburgh.

Perry L (2001) Dysphagia: the management and detection of a disabling problem. *Br J Nurs* **10**(13): 837–44

Pope JE, Curzon ME (1991) The dental status of cerebral palsied children. *Pediatr Dent* **13**(3): 156–62.

Pople J, Oliver D (1986) Oral thrush in hospice patients. *Nurs Times* **82**(45): 34–5

Richardson A (1987) A process standard for oral care. *Nurs Times* **83**(32): 38–40

Roberts A (1986) Systems of Life No.140. Senior Systems-5. *Nurs Times* **82**(33): 51–4

Roberts J (2000a) Developing an oral assessment and intervention tool for older people: 1. *Br J Nurs* **9**(17): 1124–7

Roberts J (2000b) Developing an oral assessment and intervention tool for older people: 2. *Br J Nurs* **9**(18): 2033–40

Roberts J (2000c) Developing an oral assessment and intervention tool for older people: 3. *Br J Nurs* **9**(19): 2073–8

Schweigner JL, Lang JW, Schweigner JW (1980) Oral assessment. How to do it. *Am J Nurs* **80**(4): 654–8

Scully C (2000) *The ABC of Oral Health.* BMJ Books, London

Shepherd G, Page C, Sammon P (1987) Oral hygiene. *Nurs Times* **83**(19): 25–7

Speedie G (1983) Nursology of mouth care: preventing, comforting and seeking activities related to mouth care. *J Adv Nurs* **8**: 33–40

Toghill PJ (1990) The Mouth. In: *Examining Patients: An introduction to Clinical Medicine.* Edward Arnold, London: chapter 5, 65–72

Turner G (1994) Oral care for patients who are terminally ill. *Nurs Standard* **8**(41): 49–56

Turner G (1996) Oral care. *Nurs Standard* **10**(28): 51–4

Tyldesley WR (1988) *Oral Medicine.* Wolfe Medical Publications, Ipswich

Watson (1989) Care of the mouth. *Nursing* **3**(44): 20–4

White BA (1995) The costs and consequences of neglected medically necessary oral care. *Spec Care Dentist* **15**(5): 180–6

White RJ (2000) Nurse assessment of oral health: a review of practice and education. *Br J Nurs* **9**(5): 260–6

United Kingdom Central Council for Nursing, Midwifery and Health Visiting (1992) *Code of professional conduct.* UKCC, London

2

Developing an oral assessment and intervention tool for older people

Josephine Roberts

This chapter relates to oral care for older people. The first section underlines the importance of oral assessment and evidence-based intervention of older people. It describes influences which can affect older people's ability to maintain oral healthcare practices. There is a need to examine closely issues surrounding poor oral hygiene practices and their associated ramifications for the older person. Identifying and implementing an appropriate oral assessment tool for older people should provide the foundation for the maintenance and improvement of standards of oral care practices within the clinical practice setting.

Section I

Oral care has been described as a simple but important nursing procedure, which can improve the overall well-being of patients (Bowsher *et al*, 1999). However, there is evidence that oral care (particularly in relation to oral assessment and documentation, and within the administration of oral care interventions) is often neglected or given a low priority (Hatton-Smith, 1994; Adams, 1996; Longhurst, 1998b). Where there are time constraints and/or staff shortages, oral care is often neglected (Adams, 1996).

There are also indications that nurses' knowledge of oral health problems within clinical practice is limited (Adams, 1996; Longhurst, 1998a). It has been claimed that this is due to poor oral health education in the preregistered level of nurse training (Boyle, 1992; Longhurst, 1998a; White, 2000). This can have a serious impact on the delivery of oral care to older people in the care setting.

The importance of oral care has been recognised for many years (Passos and Bland, 1966; Howarth, 1977; Maurer, 1977; Harris, 1980; Kite and Pearson, 1995; Pearson, 1996). As long ago as 1912, Marshall (cited in Passosa nd Bland, 1996) urged that, 'oral hygiene be given a high priority in the care of acutely ill patients'. Nevertheless, oral care practices have often remained rooted in tradition and ritual (Crosby, 1989; Holmes and Mountain, 1993; Hatton-Smith, 1994) rather than based on sound evidence or research (McKenna *et al*, 2000).

As a result of demographic changes, the number of older people in society is increasing (Tinker, 1997), and life expectancy is predicted to rise in the twenty-first century (Bond *et al*, 1993). In addition, older people are more likely to be dentate, ie. have some of their own natural teeth (Shay and Ship, 1995; Steele, 1996; Steele and Walls, 1997; Xavier, 2000). According to Ship (1999), this is due to increased oral health as a result of, 'advances in dental treatment, disease prevention, increased availability of dental needs'. This will obviously have an impact on the delivery of oral care for older people in clinical practice and heightens the need for professionals to assess accurately an older person's oral status on admission to a hospital or care environment so that appropriate, individualised oral care can be delivered.

The Government aims to achieve clinical effectiveness within the health service by the development of service frameworks (Department of Health [DoH], 1998). In addition, clinical governance has been introduced to monitor and raise standards of care within the clinical settings and promote evidence-based clinical practice (Brocklehurst and Walshe, 1999; King's Fund, 1999; McSherry and Haddock, 1999). Within the sphere of oral care there is a growing need to ensure that practice is based on evidence (Xavier, 2000). This has also been highlighted within the *Essence of Care* document (DoH, 2001) which is designed to raise standards, including oral care practices. The implementation of valid assessment tools and protocols of care are required to ensure that standards of oral care are of high quality.

Older people may have difficulties funding dental care where there are financial constraints (Steele, 1996), as this prevents them from attending their dentists for dental care. Being a pensioner does not entitle an older person to free dental treatment (Hardcastle, 1997). This can obviously lead some older people to neglect their dental health and omit their regular dental check-ups (Ship, 1999) which puts them at increased risk of developing dental diseases. When older people are asked how long they have had their dentures, the answer is often that they have 'had them for years' (Harrison, 1987; Griffiths and Boyle, 1993); the dentures may not have been checked since they were first made.

This indicates the need for nurses to assess accurately an older person's oral status, and identify any oral health problems in order for appropriate oral care interventions to be implemented. It also enables the nurse to give health promotion advice in relation to dental care and oral hygiene practices.

Oral diseases are mainly preventable (Ship, 1999) and therefore appropriate intervention may help prevent the incidence of oral complications and diseases.

Implications of delivering and maintaining poor oral hygiene/care

Oral health is vital for physical and emotional well-being and can have an impact on a person's quality of life (Pyle *et al*, 1998). Oral care is a basic but essential mode of intervention (Torrance, 1990; Heals, 1993; Peate, 1993) and therefore an important role for the nurse. It is vital that patients have clean and healthy mouths. Poor oral care has many associated complications.

Nutrition and hydration in relation to oral care

The oral cavity is the first part of the gastrointestinal tract, and contains the vital structures that govern one's ability to eat and drink adequately (Turner, 1996; Ship, 1999). Without appropriate oral care, patients are prone to dental and oral diseases, and these can affect eating and drinking (Simons *et al*, 1999). Dental disease can result from plaque formation and gingivitis, together with periodontal disease (Kite and Pearson, 1995). Dental caries can further damage existing teeth (Ship, 1999); this spiralling process can lead to loss of teeth together with associated discomfort and pain which can further have an impact on eating and drinking.

The presence of diseased and damaged teeth can also impair chewing (Shay and Ship, 1995), and limit the type of food that an individual is able to eat (Pettigrew, 1989). This may have a detrimental effect on an individual's diet with the consequential risk of malnutrition (Steele and Walls, 1997).

Diseases affecting the oral mucosa can create areas of inflammation and ulceration with associated pain and discomfort (Sweeney, 1998a), which can exacerbate the situation.

The presence of plaque and debris in the mouth can also affect taste. Altered taste can, in turn, affect a patient's willingness to eat and drink, which may lead to anorexia and malnutrition (Watson, 1989). Therefore, accurate oral assessment will not only assist in identifying an older person's oral hygiene needs and enable the professional to deliver appropriate intervention, but also ensure that the older person can maintain his/her nutritional and fluid intake.

Avoiding pain and promoting comfort in relation to oral care

Dental pain and discomfort are common in older people, and this can have a substantial impact on their daily lives (Steele, 1996). Healthcare professionals must provide effective oral care to assist in creating a comfortable pain-free oral cavity. Accurate assessment and appropriate, individualised oral care can help prevent oral diseases in the hospitalised patient, and therefore assists in preventing oral pain and discomfort (Xavier, 2000).

According to Hilton (1980), 'An oral problem can cause misery quite disproportionate to the size of the affected area.'

The presence of an ulcerated area or an infection can cause a great deal of pain and discomfort (Ransier *et al*, 1995) which is exacerbated when the individual is eating, drinking or talking.

Reducing risk of infection and systemic disease in relation to oral care

Oral diseases have been described as the most common disease in the world (Jones, 1998; Xavier, 2000). Poor oral hygiene is associated with numerous oral infections and diseases (Sweeney *et al*, 1995; Shay and Ship, 1995) which can be caused by fungal, viral or bacterial infections (Sweeney, 1998b), and which cause a great deal of discomfort and pain.

The presence of periodontal disease and poor oral hygiene not only have repercussions for the oral cavity (Griffiths and Boyle, 1993), but also, if untreated, perodontitis is associated with a higher incidence of coronary heart disease (DeStefano *et al*, 1993; Longhurst, 1998a). Dental infections have been linked with bacteraemia and subacute bacterial endocarditis (Peate, 1993). When there is a high density of pathogens in the oral cavity through poor oral care and a patient aspirates saliva into the lungs, the presence of these pathogens can have life-threatening consequences (Shay and Ship, 1995). Older patients are particularly at risk of developing chest infections and aspiration pneumonia (Ship, 1999).

Influence on speech in relation to oral care

An oral cavity free from infection is essential if speech is to be pain-free and effective. One of the main functions of the oral cavity is to help form speech (Shay and Ship, 1995). The presence of healthy teeth and/or well-fitting dentures also enable an older person to talk fluently, and pronounce words accurately.

A dry mouth, known as xerostomia, is a condition where there is insufficient production of saliva; this can also have an impact on speech (Ryan, 1996) and an older person's ability to communicate; they will have difficulty expressing their needs and conversing with their family.

Psychological impact in relation to oral care

The feeling of having a clean, comfortable mouth is important to us all. Good oral health can help maintain self-esteem and improve an older person's general well-being (Holmes, 1996); without adequate oral care an individual can be affected psychologically.

An individual who has been given poor oral care may have an increased build up of plaque and debris, which can produce bad breath or halitosis. Halitosis can affect an individual psychologically and develop a barrier between the patient and his/her family (Jones, 1998). A clean oral cavity has psychosocial importance and, according to Trenter Roth and Creason (1986), 'the mouth plays a major role in the physical expression of intimate affection'. The psychological impact of poor oral care must not be ignored (Barnett, 1991).

The mouth plays an important role in body image (Price, 1990; Buglass, 1995). Emphasis must be placed on allowing patients to look and feel good in themselves, particularly older people who may have other symptoms/problems.

Accountability and oral care

Accountability is a fundamental part of an individual professional's practice (Rowe, 2000); it dominates decisions made regarding all issues in health care. As a professional, one is accountable for the care delivered to patients (O'Dowd, 1998), and this includes the delivery of oral care practices. According to the UKCC (1996):

Professional accountability is fundamentally concerned with weighing up the interests of patients and clients in complex situations, using professional knowledge, judgment and skills to make a decision and enabling you to account for the decision made.

When assessing a patient's oral status and giving intervention, it is imperative to consider a patient's best interests at all times.

When exercising professional accountability, it is important to remember clause 2 of the *Code of professional conduct* (UKCC, 1992). This stipulates that nurses must, 'ensure that no action or omission on [their] part, or within [their] sphere of responsibility, is detrimental to the interests, condition or safety of patients and clients.'

It is vital for nurses to have a high level of expertise and knowledge surrounding oral care for older people to ensure that the practice is appropriate and adequate for this client group (Peate, 1993) as well as being evidence-based (Bowsher *et al*, 1999). Healthcare professionals must seek every opportunity to enhance and improve their knowledge relating to oral care practices. Without this, the professional could be at risk of litigation as a result of neglect of care (Adams, 1996).

Key points

* Oral care is a vital component in the delivery of holistic nursing care.
* There is evidence within clinical practice that the delivery of oral care is sometimes neglected and inadequate for individual patients' needs.
* Older people are increasingly likely to be dentate, highlighting the need for effective oral care.
* Written documentation to indicate oral assessment within practice is fragmented.
* Oral care interventions must be brought forward from ritualistic to evidence-based practice.

Section 2

This second section critically analyses a number of oral care agents and interventions to identify evidence-based practice relating to oral care for older people. Recommendations for practice are highlighted to guide practitioners in implementing safe and effective nursing interventions within oral care.

Numerous articles have been written by many authors about the importance of appropriate intervention in relation to oral health (Howarth, 1977; Harris, 1980; Barnett, 1991; Clarke, 1993; Jones, 1998; Bowsher *et al*, 1999; Simons *et al*, 1999; Xavier, 2000). It is impossible to examine all the methods of intervention in relation to oral care as indicated in the above literature. However, it is important to examine more closely the favoured methods used in its administration. This would assist in identifying evidence-based interventions to promote oral health for older people.

Tools and agents used in oral care interventions

Much of the previously mentioned literature contains details about using a combination of tools and interventions to administer oral care. Six practical principles have been indicated when considering the choice of oral care intervention (*Table 2.1*) (Passos and Bland, 1966).

Table 2.1: The six practical principles of oral care
Commonly handled and familiar to nurses
Readily available in hospitals
Economical to the patient/hospital
Convenient to prepare and use, in terms of the time, motion and materials required. Materials should be disposable or easily cleaned
Safe pharmacologically
Usable by a nurse without prescription by a physician

These considerations have been discussed when planning oral care (Maurer, 1977; Jenkins, 1989). However, when closely observing these principles, the authors do not consider the acceptability of the intervention for the individual patient, even though this is an important priority. It is necessary to examine more closely the following aids mentioned below in administering oral care, which are predominantly discussed in the literature.

Foam sticks

Foam sticks originated in the USA, and have become readily available in the UK for the administration of oral care since the early 1970s (Pearson, 1996). There are suggestions that the use of foam sticks to remove plaque from tooth surfaces is ineffective (Clarke, 1993; Heals, 1993; Buglass, 1995; Holmes, 1996; Pearson, 1996; Bowsher *et al*, 1999). However, the foam stick can be useful to cleanse and moisten the oral mucosa (Thurgood, 1994). They are particularly useful as a cleaning tool if the oral mucosa is fragile (Rattenbury *et al*, 1999).

There is some concern in the practice setting among fellow professionals that there is a risk of a patient biting off the foam stick and swallowing or inhaling the foam. One could, therefore, question whether there is a health and safety risk with using the foam stick for the administration of oral care. Following a review of the available literature, this does not appear to be a problem.

A swabbed-finger

A gauze swab wrapped around a gloved finger has been indicated to be an effective method of cleaning and moistening the oral mucosa (Harris, 1980). However, it is not an effective method of removing plaque and debris from tooth surfaces (Jenkins, 1989; Torrance, 1990; Heals, 1993). It has been found to compress debris and plaque into crevices and gaps in a patient's teeth exposing the individual to infections (Shepherd *et al*, 1987).

Despite this, a swabbed finger is commonly used in practice to moisten and cleanse the oral mucosa (Peate, 1993; Turner, 1996); it is also used for patients who are critically ill and where the professional feels that it is not appropriate to use a toothbrush. This method can also be used if the patient's condition fails to enable him/her to tolerate a mouthwash, ie. after suffering a stroke when swallowing may be impaired.

The use of swabs in conjunction with forceps has been found to cause trauma to the oral mucosa (Shepherd *et al*, 1987; Jenkins, 1989; Watson, 1989; Peate, 1993). It is not an appropriate tool in the administration of oral care and not recommended for use in clinical practice (Bowsher *et al*, 1999).

A toothbrush

The use of the toothbrush is indicated as the most effective method for removing plaque from tooth surfaces and maintaining healthy gums (Clarke, 1993; Thurgood, 1994; Turner, 1994; Buglass, 1995; Kite and Pearson, 1995; Steele and Walls, 1997; Jones, 1998; Rattenbury *et al*, 1999). All patients should have their own toothbrush (Sweeney, 1998c; Curzio and McCowan, 2000).

Care must be taken when cleansing oral mucosa with a normal toothbrush, as there are indications that it can cause trauma to soft tissues in the oral cavity (DeWalt, 1975; Holmes, 1996; Pearson, 1996). A soft-bristled paediatric-sized toothbrush is indicated as the safest method for cleaning the natural teeth of older people (Turner, 1994; Longhurst, 1998b; Bowsher *et al*, 1999). It can also be used to clean the tongue and other oral tissues as long as there is no evidence of mucosal irritation (Turner, 1996).

Gentle brushing of the teeth, gums and oral tissues not only cleanses the oral cavity, but also stimulates blood flow, thereby promoting good oral health (Thurgood, 1994). Teeth should be cleaned twice a day, morning and night, to maintain healthy teeth and gums (Sweeney, 1998c; Whitmyer *et al*, 1998).

The technique of brushing an older person's natural teeth is an important issue. The patient should be encouraged to use small individual strokes brushing away from the gums (Nicol *et al*, 2000). If a professional is assisting a patient with oral care, this is the method that should be carried out. Incorrect brushing technique can cause trauma and ulceration to the oral mucosa and result in pain and discomfort (Buglass, 1995).

The toothbrush does, however, have some problems. It can be difficult to hold and manipulate by older people with dexterity impairments (McCord and Stalker, 1988). It is, however, possible to involve the occupational therapist in adapting toothbrushes to enable the patient to hold and grip them more easily (Griffiths and Boyle, 1993; Hardcastle, 1997).

The ultrasonic toothbrush is very effective at removing dental plaque and is useful for older people with manual dexterity problems (Whitmyer *et al*, 1998). However, Holmes (1996) has indicated that the electric toothbrush has limited value for the removal of plaque. It is also costly which could prove to be a problem with elderly people (Griffiths and Boyle, 1993).

Lemon and glycerine swabs

The use of lemon and glycerine swabs as a tool for oral hygiene has been contraindicated because of the drying effect on the oral mucosa and the potential risk of decalcifying a patient's teeth (Buglass, 1995; Kite and Pearson, 1995; Bowsher *et al*, 1999). Lemon and glycerine swabs may initially moisten the oral mucosa, but have a drying effect if used in the long term (Foss-Durant and McAffee, 1997). Lemon can lower the oral pH to an acid environment, which can be detrimental to an older patient's teeth and increase the risk of dental caries (Poland, 1987).

Glycerine has the potential to absorb moisture from the oral mucosa and dehydrates by its osmotic action, causing reflux exhaustion of the salivation process (Gooch, 1985; Buglass, 1995). Lemon and glycerine swabs are not recommended in the administration of oral care (Bowsher *et al*, 1999).

Toothpaste

Fluoride toothpaste, used in combination with a soft toothbrush, represents the most effective cleaning agent to maintain clean and healthy teeth (Turner, 1996; Rattenbury *et al*, 1999). Fluoride helps to strengthen the enamel surface giving the tooth more resistance to dental diseases (Griffiths and Boyle, 1993). However, when using a toothpaste it is important to remove all traces of the toothpaste from the oral cavity as it can have a drying effect on the mouth (Gooch, 1985). Prolonged presence of toothpaste on the oral mucosa can have a burning effect (Turner, 1994).

It is important to use only a small amount of toothpaste, which should be pressed into the surface of the toothbrush (Jones, 1998). This will avoid particles of toothpaste coming away from the toothbrush surface and being left in the oral cavity. This is an important issue in older people who might find it difficult to rinse their mouths adequately because of poor oral dexterity.

Lip lubricant

A lip lubricant is an accepted way to prevent the drying and cracking of older persons' lips (Turner, 1994; Bowsher *et al*, 1999). Petroleum jelly (Vaseline) appears to be the most effective agent used for the lips of older people (Heals, 1993; Bowsher *et al*, 1999). This, as well as an emollient, is widely used in the clinical practice setting, and is particularly beneficial for patients who have a poor oral fluid intake and are at risk of developing dry lips.

Mouthwashes and gargles

A mouthwash rinses and moistens the oral cavity (Jenkins, 1989). There are numerous mouthwash preparations, which can cause confusion when treating older people. To attempt to clarify issues pertaining to oral preparations, it is important to examine some of the most commonly used products in more detail.

Chlorhexidine

Many antiseptic mouthwashes are available under prescription which, 'apart from those containing chlorhexidine gluconate, are of limited value as they have only a transient effect' (Jones, 1998). Chlorhexidine mouthwash is effective for plaque control and for its antibacterial and fungicidal properties (Griffiths and Boyle, 1993; Heals, 1993; Jones, 1998; Sweeney, 1998c; Bowsher *et al*, 1999; Rattenbury *et al*, 1999; Curzio and McCowan, 2000 and *Chapter 3*). It, therefore, can play an important role in inhibiting the development of oral infections (Gooch, 1985; Barnett, 1991; Thurgood, 1994).

Corsodyl, which contains chlorhexidine gluconate, appears to be appropriate for use as an aid to mechanical cleansing in oral hygiene, particularly for older people who have difficulty cleaning their own teeth because of dexterity problems (Griffiths and Boyle, 1993). It is a useful adjunct to oral care (Xavier, 2000). Corsodyl comes in the form of mouthwash, dental gel and oral spray and therefore is versatile in its use (*British National Formulary [BNF]*, 2000).

With long-term use, chlorhexidine can stain the teeth (Barnett, 1991; Hatton-Smith, 1994; Thurgood, 1994; Gibson, 1999/2000) and cause dis-colouration of the tongue (Heals, 1993; Turner, 1996). There is indication that oral antiseptics may cause mucosal irritation (Turner, 1996; Gibson, 1999/ 2000). They can also disrupt the normal flora in the oral cavity and should not be overused (Barnett, 1991; Holmes, 1996). Chlorhexidine gluconate can be diluted before use as a mouthwash to make it easy to tolerate for patients (Turner, 1996).

Hydrogen peroxide

Hydrogen peroxide has been used as an effective oral cleansing agent through its ability to destroy chemically bacteria, and the mechanical action of removing debris to cleanse wound surfaces in the oral cavity (Passos and Bland, 1966; Maurer, 1977). However, hydrogen peroxide can have a detrimental effect on fresh granulating surfaces in the oral cavity as it tends to break down the new tissue (Passos and Bland, 1966; Gooch, 1985; Thurgood, 1994).

The foaming effect of hydrogen peroxide within the oral cavity can potentially be dangerous in patients who have impaired cough reflex (Thurgood, 1994). Hydrogen peroxide has been found to cause abnormal change in the oral mucosa of healthy individuals and it should not be used for the administration of oral care within clinical practice (Tombes and Gallucci, 1993).

Pineapple

The use of unsweetened pineapple as an aid for oral care has been indicated in some of the literature (Hilton, 1980; Heals, 1993; Regnard *et al*, 1997; Rattenbury *et al*, 1999). According to Regnard *et al* (1997), 'a coated tongue can be cleared in days with the proteolytic enzyme annanase, effectively delivered by regular chewing of unsweetened pineapple chunks'. This is difficult to implement within clinical practice because many older people find pineapple chunks difficult to chew. However, fresh pineapple juice may be a possibility, and should be considered for patients who might benefit from it.

There is evidence that other fresh fruit and fruit juices can be effective in freshening the oral cavity and relieving a dry mouth (Heals, 1993). This should be encouraged in clinical practice, not only because of the benefits for the oral mucosa but also to help older people's nutritional status (Eliopoulos, 1997). However, too much fruit juice, which has a high acid content, can erode the tooth enamel; therefore, fruit juice consumption should be regulated (Griffiths and Boyle, 1993).

Saliva substitutes

The use of saliva substitutes for the relief of xerostomia has been indicated as having some benefits (Thurgood, 1994; Bowsher *et al*, 1999). Saliva substitutes can be particularly useful for patients with persistent or chronic dry mouths (Griffiths and Boyle, 1993). Saliva substitutes are intended to resemble natural saliva and mainly come in the form of an oral spray (Thurgood, 1994; *BNF*, 2000).

However, for their maximum benefit, a saliva substitute should be used correctly (Ryan, 1996). The saliva substitute glandosane is reported to last one to two hours (Heals, 1993). According to Ryan (1996):

> *When using one of the spray formulations, the upper and lower surfaces of the tongue and the sides of the mouth must all be coated, and the application repeated at regular intervals*

Ideally, for maximum affect, patients should be taught how to administer a saliva substitute independently (Ryan, 1996). This can only be possible if the older person has the ability to operate a small spray appliance, and is cognitively able to undertake this procedure unaided. If this is not possible, the professional must then assist the patient.

Unfortunately, saliva substitutes do not have the protective properties of natural saliva (Buglass, 1995; Holmes, 1996). It is, therefore, important for the professional to consider that if an older person is having a saliva substitute administered, he/she could be at further risk of developing oral complications.

There is evidence that administering frequent sips of plain cold water are as effective as a saliva substitute (Regnard *et al*, 1997). Therefore, one should ensure before recommending an expensive saliva substitute, that frequent oral fluids are offered to the older patient suffering from xerostomia to see if this helps relieve his/her symptoms. The importance of encouraging an older person to drink plenty of fluids cannot be overemphasised. This can provide great relief for a dry mouth and keep the oral mucosa hydrated and lubricated (Heals, 1993).

Sodium bicarbonate

Sodium bicarbonate has been found to be an effective oral cleansing agent (Howarth, 1977; Hatton-Smith, 1994; Buglass, 1995). It is found to dissolve mucus and loosen stagnated food particles and other debris present in the oral cavity (Maurer, 1977). It is also recommended to be used when tenacious mucous is present or there are crusted areas present in the mouth (Rattenbury *et al*, 1999).

However, there is evidence that sodium bicarbonate can cause superficial burns to the oral mucosa if the agent is not diluted correctly (Crosby, 1989; Heals, 1993; Kite and Pearson, 1995). Sodium bicarbonate solution is alkaline and can alter the oral pH allowing bacteria to multiply, thus upsetting the normal oral flora (DeWalt and Haines, 1969; Crosby, 1989; Kite and Pearson, 1995). There is indication that sodium bicarbonate, when used as an oral cleansing agent, is unpleasant to the taste (Bowsher *et al*, 1999).

After the above issues are considered, there is evidence to suggest that sodium bicarbonate, used as an oral cleanser, should be used with great care and only if other methods have not been effective.

Sodium chloride

Sodium chloride can be used as an effective oral cleanser (Griffiths and Boyle, 1993); as a 0.9% solution it is economic and safe to use (Maurer, 1977; Gooch, 1985). Sodium chloride is naturally found in the body and can be safely used as a mouthwash (Jenkins, 1989). There is some indication that sodium chloride can promote healing and formation of granulating tissue (Turner, 1996). Where there is evidence of swollen and painful gums, a warm salt solution can alleviate these symptoms (Speedie, 1983).

There is limited sound evidence for the use of sodium chloride as an agent used in oral hygiene. Bowsher *et al* (1999) indicate that there is insufficient evidence for its use within clinical practice. It is evident that further research is necessary before sodium chloride is readily used as an oral agent.

Thymol preparations

There is some confusion with regard to the different thymol mouthwash preparations from the available literature. For example, they are referred to as glycothymoline (Howarth, 1977; Gooch, 1985; Barnett, 1991; Buglass, 1995; Nicol *et al*, 2000), thymol (Hatton-Smith, 1994), and glycerin thymol (Heals, 1993; Rattenbury *et al*, 1999).

Thymol mouthwash tablets are used readily within clinical practice even though this may not be at the request of the patient. It is also evident in clinical practice that the mouthwash tablets are not always diluted according to the manufacturer's instructions, ie. one tablet in a tumbler-full of water.

The literature indicates that thymol or glycothymoline mouthwashes have no actual benefits (Barnett, 1991; Heals, 1993; Rattenbury *et al*, 1999). Used on its own, this form of mouthwash has no cleansing properties for the oral cavity (Rattenbury *et al*, 1999). It has an initial refreshing action, but no lasting affect (Nicol *et al*, 2000), and can leave an unpleasant taste in the patient's mouth after frequent use (Hatton-Smith, 1994). The use of a thymol mouthwash agent must, therefore, be questioned and used with caution. Patient choice should be a factor in its use.

Water

The use of water has been undervalued in oral care, but it is a safe and economical agent to use for cleansing and moistening the oral cavity (Jenkins, 1989; Torrance, 1990; Clarke, 1993). Water, which has a short action, can also be used as an effective mouthwash (Clarke, 1993; Hatton-Smith, 1994; Bowsher *et al*, 1999; Nicol *et al*, 2000). Water has a pH of 7, similar to saliva, which has a pH of between 6.8 and 7 (Gooch, 1985).

As water is the ideal pH for the oral cavity, one could argue that it is the natural agent to be used for oral hygiene (Speedie, 1983). It causes minimal disruption to normal oral flora to maintain a healthy oral mucosa (Clarke, 1993). Water can be used in conjunction with a soft toothbrush and fluoride toothpaste to clean tooth surfaces and oral mucosa. As water is so readily available and economical to use, it is appropriate to use it in conjunction with other oral care utensils.

Care of dentures

The care of dentures, too often neglected, is an important part of oral management (McCord and Stalker, 1988; Heals, 1993). Mistakes can arise in failing to identify the presence of dentures on a patient's admission (Longhurst, 1998a, b), thus not removing them for normal cleansing. This highlights the need for careful oral assessment when an older person is first admitted to hospital.

Individual patients' knowledge of how to care adequately for their own dentures is sometimes lacking (Jagger and Harrison, 1995). This demonstrates the need for the professional to educate older people in the care of their dentures and to promote independence in so doing.

Part of the care of dentures should involve encouraging an older person to remove his/her dentures after each meal and rinsing them under cold water to remove debris (Griffiths and Boyle, 1993). Food particles tend to become attached and accumulate on denture surfaces; the normal cleansing action of the oral cavity is not sufficient to remove all debris (McCord and Stalker, 1988).

Dentures should be removed at night and cleaned using cold water and a denture brush or toothbrush with hand soap or washing-up detergent (Clarke, 1993; Griffiths and Boyle, 1993; Xavier, 2000). Toothpaste should not be used as it can damage the denture surface (Clarke, 1993). Dentures should not be left to dry out or come in contact with hot water as this can warp the denture, thus changing its shape (Shepherd *et al*, 1987). Following careful cleansing, dentures should be left out to soak at night in a suitable denture-cleansing agent.

It is important to remember that individual dentures are made out of different materials and it would be appropriate for patients to use there own denture-cleansing agent; if the wrong cleansing agent is used the denture surface could become damaged (Harrison, 1987; Jagger and Harrison, 1995). The importance of removing dentures at night should be emphasised when promoting independence; failing to do so can make an older person susceptible to developing denture stomatitis (Sweeney, 1998c).

Conclusions

After reviewing the available literature it is evident that no single intervention is appropriate for all patients (Speedie, 1983; Holmes, 1996). This must be considered when assessing and developing a plan of care for patients. The use of a toothbrush, toothpaste and water are the favoured tools and agents that individuals would normally use at home for their own natural teeth (Clarke, 1993). Therefore, it would be appropriate for them to use the same utensils while in hospital. This would also be more pleasant for the patient and would comply with Passos and Bland's (1966) practical principles when choosing an oral care intervention.

It is also important to remember that each individual has his/her own standards of oral hygiene and this should be considered when assisting with oral care (Pearson, 1996). When choosing an oral intervention, it is vital to enable the patient to have choice in what oral care method is used. Patients should be encouraged to be independent with their own oral hygiene practices wherever possible (Sweeney, 1998c). This assists in facilitating older people's independence in relation to their own oral care. It also gives them an element of self-empowerment which is so vital in healthcare delivery (Wilkinson and Miers, 1999).

Key points

- ⌘ Oral care is often a ritualistic area of practice based on tradition.
- ⌘ The care of dentures is an aspect of care that is all too often neglected.
- ⌘ There is a need to ensure that oral care interventions are evidence-based to provide a high standard of oral care for older people.
- ⌘ No single intervention is appropriate for all patients; however, the toothbrush, toothpaste and water are the most favoured methods to keep natural teeth healthy.

Section 3

The third section looks at the factors which have an impact on oral health, and which must be considered when assessing a patient's oral health status. The correlation between holistic assessment and careful documentation is examined, together with its associated relationship with maintaining effective oral care. This section also critiques a collection of published oral assessment tools to identify whether they would be appropriate for rehabilitation client groups. After identifying the lack of a suitable oral assessment tool within the literature, the need to develop an appropriate one is addressed. An oral assessment and intervention tool which has been developed in the author's clinical area is outlined.

Accurate documentation through assessment should be a vital form of communication among healthcare professionals and is necessary for good general practice. In relation to assessment and intervention, accurate documentation and record keeping is an integral part of care delivery (UKCC, 1993). Accurate nursing documentation is of paramount importance, and aids a pathway to ensure that high standards of care are delivered to patients (Bernick and Richards, 1994). Oral assessment and documentation should provide the basis for oral care interventions.

Assessment is the first step and a fundamental part of the nursing process (Eliopoulos, 1997). According to Ryrie and Edwards (1999), 'Assessment is a cornerstone of high-quality care upon which all subsequent interventions are based.' It is a process of gathering vital and accurate information to provide a baseline to enable decisions to be made about the patient's care (Heath, 2000). This helps to provide a pathway in offering people high standards of patient-focused care in relation to their oral health requirements. Assessment should have a holistic focus. This is particularly important for older people who can have multiple pathological problems (RCN, 2000b). These include reduced visual acuity and psychomotor skills and physical impairments, which can reduce an older person's ability to attend to his/her own oral hygiene (Walls, 1996).

Factors to consider when assessing an older person's oral status

When assessing an older patient's oral health many factors must be considered.

The oral cavity

This can have an impact on oral health (Shay and Ship, 1995). It includes the condition of existing teeth and dentures and also the condition of oral mucosa, gingiva and periodontium (Griffiths and Boyle, 1993). The presence of dental plaque, which only takes about twenty-four hours to develop, is detrimental to dental health (Clarke, 1993).

Diet and fluids

Taken by mouth these have an impact on the condition of the oral cavity and subsequent oral health (Barnett, 1991; Heals, 1993). A reduced dietary and fluid intake and associated dehydration can have a disastrous effect on the oral cavity (Barnett, 1991; Clarke, 1993). Deficiencies in certain vitamins, eg. vitamins B and C, can have an impact on oral health (Gooch, 1985; Griffiths and Boyle, 1993).

Intake of certain drugs

Certain drugs have an impact on the oral mucosa (Adams, 1996), eg. the administration of chemotherapy (Beck, 1979; Richardson, 1987; Eilers *et al*, 1988; Crosby, 1989). Patients who are taking antibiotics and steroids are more prone to oral infections (Sweeney, 1998b). Many medications taken by older people can reduce the production of saliva, causing xerostomia (Torrance, 1990; Ship, 1999), eg. antidepressants, antihypertensives and diuretics (Shay and Ship, 1995). Drugs, including aspirin and iron preparations, can cause ulceration if left in contact with the oral mucosa too long and not swallowed correctly (Sweeney, 1998a).

Underlying medical conditions

These can predispose to oral complications (Griffiths and Boyle, 1993). An example of this is diabetes, which has been known to increase the incidence of periodontal disease (Shay and Ship, 1995). Incidences of oral candidiasis infections are more likely in patients with diabetes (Soames and Southam, 1998). Iron deficiency anaemia greatly increases the incidence of persistent oral ulceration, generalised soreness of the oral cavity with increased incidence of oral infections (Griffiths and Boyle, 1993).

Oxygen administration and mouth breathers

These patients are more likely to develop a dry oral mucosa with subsequent cracking, which facilitates infection (Hatton-Smith, 1994).

Older people

The ageing process may cause alterations in the oral cavity (Holmes, 1996; White, 2000). These include reduced salivary production, tooth structure changes due to wear and tear, and increasing prevalence of dental problems (Barnett, 1991; Walls, 1996). There is also a change in the condition of the oral cavity in general with mucosal atrophy and thinning (Ship, 1999). This can greatly increase the incidence of oral ulceration and associated infection (Holmes, 1996).

Manual dexterity

These problems can reduce the likelihood of older patients being able to manipulate a toothbrush effectively to clean their teeth adequately (Pettigrew, 1989). This can put them at an increased risk of dental caries and periodontal disease.

Altered levels of consciousness

These can affect an older person's oral dexterity and swallowing and, therefore, put them at risk of developing oral complications. Patients who suffer from a stroke may have difficulty clearing their mouths of debris after meals and pool food in the weak side of their mouth (Griffiths and Boyle, 1993; Longhurst, 1998b). This can further put them at risk of developing oral infections.

Poor cognitive function

Older people with poor cognitive function may forget the need to clean their teeth regularly. This could put them at a greater risk of developing oral complications. The incidence of depression is increased in the older age group (Barder *et al*, 1994). Associated with depression is the incidence of apathy and listlessness, which could result in self-neglect. This may affect personal oral hygiene and hence increases the risk of oral complications (Whitton, 1994; Sweeney, 1999).

The factors that can influence oral health and have an impact on the older person's overall condition directly or indirectly are described as 'risk factors' (Jenkins, 1989; Clarke, 1993; Walls, 1996; White, 2000; Xavier, 2000).

Identifying an appropriate oral assessment tool for practice

The importance of oral assessment has been highlighted by numerous authors (eg. Jenkins, 1989; Boyle, 1992; Holmes and Mountain, 1993; Turner, 1994; Rattenbury *et al*, 1999; Xavier, 2000).

To identify an oral assessment tool for an elderly client rehabilitation group, it is necessary to review and analyse a few existing tools, which are currently available in the literature. Many of the oral assessment tools described in the literature are targeted at acutely ill patients either undergoing chemotherapy or in intensive care.

Passos and Bland (1966) devised an oral assessment guide to calculate by a numerical rating scale the effectiveness of three oral hygiene agents used for acutely ill surgical patients. A study in an elderly client group was conducted to identify the effects of using either a toothbrush or a 'toothette' (pink foam stick) on the oral mucosa (DeWalt, 1975). In this study, a numerical rating scale was used which was based on the discussed rating scale (Passos and Bland, 1966). Neither of these oral rating scales indicated that they were used as an oral assessment guide, other than identifying the effects of oral agents on the oral mucosa.

Eilers *et al* (1988) developed an oral assessment tool which was used to identify oral cavity change in a sample receiving cancer treatment. The tool was based on clinical experience undertaken by the researchers and supported by a review of available literature.

A review of previously published assessment tools (*Table 2.2*) identified areas in the oral cavity that had been indicated as important areas to assess. The oral assessment guide identified eight categories to be assessed, and three numerical and descriptive ratings which are scored to determine the condition of the oral cavity. This is based on a continuum scale, from the best to the worst scenario, while observing the oral cavity as indicated by the researchers.

A pilot study was undertaken to test the oral assessment tool developed (Eilers *et al*, 1988) for usability. This provided evidence to indicate how effective the tool would be in clinical practice. Twenty subjects were used in the convenience sample of patients undergoing bone marrow transplantation.

The oral assessment tool did not consider the additional 'at risk' factors which affect oral health as previously indicated in the text. These could include various factors, eg. the patient's age, his/her oral intake, any underlying medical condition, the patient's cognitive function, details of drugs taken and the patient's physical condition.

The oral assessment tool was specifically targeted for a specialist group undergoing treatment for cancer (Eilers *et al*, 1988). This, together with the above mentioned factors, would therefore limit its use for rehabilitation patients.

Jenkins (1989) reflects on his own previous experience of working in an intensive care unit (ITU), and identifies patients who are 'at risk' of developing oral complications and diseases. His findings stress the need for an 'at risk' calculator to assess patients' requirements in relation to oral intervention. Jenkins undertook the development of an oral calculator based on Norton *et al*'s (1962) scale, to indicate the risk of pressure sore prevention. It identified five 'at risk' categories which included the patient's age, normal oral condition, mastication ability, and nutritional and airway status. A rating scale of one to four gives an indication of the condition of each category. Each category is then added up to give a total score to indicate the level of intervention required. Additional risk factors are highlighted, which should be added to the final score.

The scoring to indicate levels of intervention, range from one-hourly to two-hourly care. Obviously, it is appropriate in an ITU setting to provide this level of intervention; however, in a rehabilitation unit for older people it would not be appropriate to undertake this on every patient. Part of the role of a professional is to encourage and support patients to regain their independence.

The oral calculator developed by Jenkins (1989) does not assess the patient's oral cavity adequately. It allows the examiner to identify whether the condition of the oral cavity is good, fair, poor or very poor. These categories are extremely vague, and it is questionable how one would define them. Therefore, one could question the calculator's reliability. The oral calculator has limitations because it does not allow the examiner to assess the oral cavity in detail, and many oral problems/diseases may be accidentally missed.

Rattenbury *et al* (1999) developed an oral assessment tool combined with suggested nursing care for inpatients in their local hospital. According to the researchers, the oral assessment tool is 'user-friendly'. For an oral assessment tool to be utilised in the practice areas, it is important for it to be quick and easy to use; anything too complicated tends to get either not used, or inadequately completed.

Rattenbury *et al* (1999) included six areas of the oral cavity to assess (*Table 2.2*). However, the researchers have not included the patients' swallowing and voice as areas for assessment; these have been highlighted in many of the above articles as important areas to assess.

The oral assessment tool also does not include the 'at risk' areas that previous authors have highlighted as important factors to consider when assessing a patient's oral status (Jenkins, 1989; Clarke, 1993; Griffiths and Boyle, 1993; White, 2000). These 'at risk' factors can make an individual more prone to developing oral health problems as discussed previously.

The authors have not included in their oral assessment tool any areas for a registered nurse to write in each assessment area, ie. a column could be useful to indicate why the areas to be examined are problem areas. One could question why the authors have not included a referral to the dentist in the suggested nursing care column, eg. if a patient's teeth are causing difficulty with eating it may be appropriate to refer him/her to a dentist rather than a doctor. Many authors have highlighted the importance of using a dentist in oral care (Griffiths and Boyle, 1993; Sweeney, 1998c; White, 2000).

Discussion

After studying the available literature in depth, it is possible to identify that there are no oral assessment tools specifically targeted at an older client group undergoing rehabilitation. However, elderly people are 'at risk' of developing oral health problems (Jenkins, 1989; Clarke, 1993; White, 2000). Griffiths and Boyle (1993) indicate that those who are 'at risk' are the patients with special needs, ie. those with physical disability, who are medically compromised and who are dependent. One could also argue that many older people fall into one or more of these categories.

Table 2.2: Studies on the assessment of oral care

Reference	Year	Lips	Tongue	Saliva	Voice	Teeth/dentures	Mucous membranes	Gingiva	Swallow
Passos and Bland	1966	*	*	*		*	*		
DeWalt	1975	*	*	*		*	*	*	
Maurer	1977	*	*	*		*		*	
Beck	1979	*	*	*	*	*	*	*	*
Eilers et al	1988	*	*	*	*	*	*	*	*
Heals	1993	*	*	*		*	*		
Jenkins	1989†								
Turner	1994	*	*	*	*	*	*	*	*
Jones	1988	*	*			*	*	*	
Rattenbury et al	1999	*	*	*		*	*	*	
White	2000	*	*	*		*	*	*	
Xavier	2000	*	*			*	*	*	

* The need for the category in question to be assessed

† The Jenkins' oral calculator examines five categories: the patient's age, the normal oral condition, the mastication ability, the nutritional state and the airway. It also examines whether the patient is taking large-dose antibiotics/steroid therapy, is suffering from diabetes mellitus, has a low haemoglobin or is immunosuppressed

The importance of accurate oral assessment to provide the administration of appropriate oral care interventions has been highlighted. Through direct observation in clinical practice, it is evident that a more structured approach for oral assessment is necessary.

From observations in clinical practice there is little evidence to indicate that oral assessment is taking place. There is, therefore, a particular need for a systematic oral assessment tool to facilitate the documentation of older people's oral status when they are admitted to the rehabilitation unit.

It is not possible to review and critique all the available oral assessment tools contained in the literature. However, it is clear that there is no oral assessment tool currently specifically suitable for a rehabilitative environment focusing on older people. With this in mind, one has to consider developing a tool suitable for the client group in question.

The available literature does give an indication of particular areas on which to focus in relation to assessing an older person's oral status (*Table 2.2*).

Once an oral assessment has been undertaken, it is vital for appropriate intervention to be implemented. The oral assessment and intervention tool devised for use within the author's own clinical area is shown in *Figure 2.1*. While developing the tool, it was vital to consider the contents of previous literature reviews and research articles, and to use the material available to ensure a high content reliability. It was also important to use a multidisciplinary approach and involve other professionals, eg. dental practitioners, occupational therapists and speech therapists (White, 2000). This is particularly important in a rehabilitation setting where interdisciplinary team working is the philosophy of care.

Before developing the oral assessment and intervention tool, it was important to obtain feedback and information from other nursing professionals. This was achieved by the use of a questionnaire, which was completed by senior nursing colleagues (*Table 2.3*).

Table 2.3: Mouth care questionnaire

1. How frequently should we assess our patients' oral cavity?
2. How frequently should we evaluate our patients' oral cavity?
3. How frequently should we encourage our patients to clean their teeth/dentures if they are independent?
4. What level of intervention/mouth care would you feel was necessary to give to patients who are suffering from the following: unconscious; semi-conscious; and have swallowing difficulties?
5. What would you like to see included in an oral assessment tool?

Once the oral assessment and intervention tool had been developed, it was necessary to implement it into clinical practice gradually and to give all trained and untrained nursing staff tuition in how to use it. The tool was initially piloted and used for all new patients admitted to the ward. It was therefore possible to monitor closely its use and enable staff to become familiar with its use.

Name:		Hospital number:	Ward:	
What is your normal mouth care routine at home? When did you last see a dentist?				
Assessment — use tongue compressor		**Circle Y or N**		**Suggested nursing care**
Lips	Dry/cracked	Y	N	Apply an emollient, petroleum gel or Vaseline
Tongue	Dry/coated?	Y	N	Clean with soft toothbrush and tooth-paste. Offer frequent fluids and fruit juices
	Evidence of ulceration/ soreness?	Y	N	Refer to doctor. Use monitoring goal to document intervention requirements
Saliva	Dry mouth? (xerostomia)	Y	N	Offer frequent fluids and/or iced water. Offer mouthwash. If symptoms persistent refer to doctor for saliva substitute
Teeth	Own teeth?	Y	N	Encourage independence with cleaning teeth night and morning. Use soft toothbrush and toothpaste
	Evidence of plaque/debris?	Y	N	Supervise with oral care. Use soft toothbrush and toothpaste
Dentures	Top denture? Lower denture? Dentures and own teeth?	Y Y Y	N N N	Encourage independence with cleaning dentures night and morning with soap and water; rinse dentures after meals. Clean teeth as above. Remove dentures at night and leave to soak
Pain	When eating/ drinking caused by teeth/dentures	Y	N	Refer to dentist
Gums/soft tissue	Evidence of sore-ness/ulceration	Y	N	Refer to doctor. Use monitoring goal to document intervention requirements
Swallowing	Difficulty with swallowing?	Y	N	Clean teeth and/or dentures and oral cavity after each meal. Refer to speech therapist
Nutrition	Fluid/dietary intake poor? Dehydrated?	Y	N	Offer hourly fluids. May require hourly mouth care. Use monitoring goal if appropriate
Speech difficulty	Due to dry mouth	Y	N	Offer frequent fluids (see above). Refer to dentist
Dexterity problems	Having difficulty holding tooth-brush?	Y	N	Refer to OT for toothbrush adaptations. May need supervision with mouth care
Cognitive problems	Evidence of short-term memory loss and/or confusion	Y	N	May need supervision with mouth care

Figure 2.1: Oral assessment and intervention tool

It was also important to obtain feedback from staff members on the oral assessment and intervention tool. This helps to facilitate ownership and involves them in the tool's development, which is vital when making any changes in clinical practice. Generally, the tool was found to be quick and easy to complete and gave nursing staff an indication as to what interventions were required. The oral intervention protocol gives advice on oral care practice. This can easily be used for healthcare assistants (HCA), who give most of the oral care to inpatients within clinical practice.

Conclusion

Developing and implementing an oral assessment and intervention tool for use in clinical practice supports a quality mechanism, which maintains and improves standards of care (RCN, 2000a). It can also provide the evidence-based intervention in relation to oral care practice that is required within the clinical governance framework to give quality health care (McSherry and Haddock, 1999). The tool is also now being implemented within a palliative care setting for older people with complex nursing needs. The tool has been found to be extremely valuable and reliable to assess patients oral health status. It also gives a framework for oral care practices.

It is recommended that different clinical settings use an oral assessment tool relevant to their client group. Assessment needs to guide intervention that is evidence-based. The assessment and intervention tool now being developed within the clinical area, using rigorous research, enables the development of a valid and reliable assessment tool. To further develop the tool, it will later be tested and used in other inpatient areas for similar client groups within the trust.

Key points

⌘ There are numerous factors to consider when assessing an older person's oral health.

⌘ A thorough, holistic oral assessment through accurate documentation is vital to effective oral care.

⌘ There are many oral assessment tools but they are not applicable for older people undergoing rehabilitation.

⌘ A simple but effective oral assessment and intervention tool is demonstrated and is now being piloted in practice.

References

Adams R (1996) Qualified nurses lack adequate knowledge related to oral health, resulting in inadequate oral care of patients on medical wards. *J Adv Nurs* **24**(3): 552–60

Barder L, Slimmer L, Lesage J (1994) Depression and issues of control among elderly people in health care settings. *J Adv Nurs* **20**(4): 597–604

Barnett J (1991) A reassessment of oral health care. *Prof Nurse* **6**(12): 703–8

Beck S (1979) Impact of a systematic oral care protocol on stomatitis after chemotherapy. *Cancer Nurs* **2**(3): 185–9

Bernick L, Richards P (1994) Nursing documentation: a program to promote and sustain improvement. *J Contin Educ Nurs* **25**(5): 203–8

Bond J, Coleman P, Peace S (1993) *Ageing in Society: An Introduction to Social Gerontology*. 2nd edn. Sage, London

Boyle S (1992) Assessing mouth care. *Nurs Times* **88**(15): 44–6

Bowsher J, Boyle S, Griffiths J (1999) Oral care. *Nurs Standard* **13**(37): 31

BNF (2000) *British National Formulary*. Royal Pharmaceutical Society of Great Britain, London

Brocklehurst N, Walshe K (1999) Quality and the new NHS. *Nurs Standard* **13**(51): 46–53

Buglass EA (1995) Oral hygiene. *Br J Nurs* **4**(9): 516–19

Clarke G (1993) Mouth care and the hospitalized patient. *Br J Nurs* **2**(4): 225–7

Crosby C (1989) Method in mouth care. *Nurs Times* **85**(35): 38–41

Curzio J, McCowan M (2000) Getting research into practice: developing oral hygiene standards. *Br J Nurs* **9**(7): 434–8

Department of Health (1998) *A First Class Service: Quality in the New NHS*. DOH, London

Department of Health (2001) *The Essence of Care. Patient-focused benchmarking for healthcare practitioners*. DoH, London

DeStefano F, Anda RF, Kahn HS, Williamson DF, Russell CM (1993) Dental disease and risk of coronary heart disease and mortality. *Br Med J* **306**: 688–91

DeWalt EM (1975) Effects of timed hygiene measures on oral mucosa in a group of elderly subjects. *Nurs Res* **24**(2): 104–8

DeWalt EM, Haines A (1969) The effects of specific stressors on healthy oral mucosa. *Nurs Res* **18**(1): 22–7

Eilers J, Berger AM, Petersen MC (1988) Development, testing, and application of the oral assessment guide. *Oncol Nurse Forum* **15**(3): 325–30

Eliopoulos C (1997) *Gerontological Nursing*. 4th edn. Lippincott-Raven, New York

Foss-Durant AM, McAffee A (1997) A comparison of three oral care products commonly used in practice. *Clin Nurs Res* **6**(1): 90–104

Gibson J (1999/2000) Medications for oral soft tissue diseases. *J Nurs Care* **2**(4): 7–10

Gooch J (1985) Mouth care. *Prof Nurse* **1**(3): 77–8

Griffiths J, Boyle S (1993) *Colour Guide to Holistic Oral Care: A Practical Approach*. Mosby, London

Hardcastle K (1997) Promoting oral health in older people. *Nurs Times* **93**(30): 56–7

Harris MD (1980) Tools for mouth care. *Nurs Times* **76**(8): 340–2

Harrison (1987) Denture care. *Nurs Times* **83**(19): 28–9

Hatton-Smith CK (1994) A last bastion of ritualized practice? A review of nurses' knowledge of oral healthcare. *Prof Nurse* **9**(5): 304–8

Heals D (1993) A key to wellbeing. Oral hygiene in patients with advanced cancer. *Prof Nurse* **8**(6): 391–8

Heath H (2000) The nurse's role in assessing an older person. *Elderly Care* **12**(1): 23–4

Hilton D (1980) Oral hygiene and infection. *Nurs Times* **76**: 1270–1

Holmes S (1996) Nursing management of oral care in older patients. *Nurs Times* **92**(9): 37–9

Holmes S, Mountain E (1993) Assessment of oral status: evaluation of three oral assessment guides. *J Clin Nurs* **2**: 35–40

Howarth H (1977) Mouth care procedures for the very ill. *Nurs Times* **73**: 354–7

Jagger DC, Harrison A (1995) Denture cleansing — the best approach. *Br Dental J* **178**: 413–17

Jenkins D (1989) Oral care in the ICU: an important nursing role. *Nurs Standard* **4**(7): 24–8

Jones CV (1998) The importance of oral hygiene in nutritional support. *Br J Nurs* **7**(2): 74–83

King's Fund (1999) Clinical governance. *Nurs Standard* **13**(28): 31–2

Kite K, Pearson L (1995) A rationale for mouth care: the integration of theory with practice. *Int Crit Care Nurs* **11**(2): 71–6

Longhurst RH (1998a) A cross-sectional study of the oral healthcare instruction given to nurses during their basic training. *Br Dent J* **184**(9): 453–7

Longhurst R (1998b) Down in the mouth. *Nurs Times* **94**(46): 24–5

Maurer J (1977) Providing optimal oral care. *Nurs Clin North Am* **12**(4): 671–85

McKenna H, Cutliffe J, McKenna P (2000) Evidence-based practice: demolishing some myths. *Nurs Standard* **14**(16): 39–42

McCord F, Stalker A (1988) Brushing up on oral care. *Nurs Times* **84**(13): 40–1

McSherry R, Haddock J (1999) Evidence-based health care: its place within clinical governance. *Br J Nurs* **8**(2): 113–16

Marshall JS (1912) *Mouth Hygiene and Mouth Sepsis*. JP Lippincott, Philadelphia

Maurer J (1977) Providing optimal care. *Nurs Clin North Am* **12**(4): 671–85

Nicol M, Bavin C, Bedford-Turner S, Cronin P, Rawlings-Anderson K (2000) *Essential Nursing Skills*. Mosby Harcourt, London: 199–201

Norton D, Exton-Smith A, McLaren R (1962) *An Investigation of Geriatric Nursing Problems in Hospital. National Corporation for the Care of Old People* (Reprinted 1975). Churchill Livingstone, Edinburgh

O'Dowd A (1998) Nurse training fails oral exam. *Nurs Times* **94**(46): 25

Passos JY, Bland LM (1966) Effects of agents used for oral hygiene. *Nurs Res* **15**(3): 196–202

Pearson LS (1996) A comparison of the ability of foam swabs and toothbrushes to remove dental plaque: implications for nursing practice. *J Adv Nurs* **23**(1): 62–9

Peate I (1993) Nurse-administered oral hygiene in the hospitalized patient. *Br J Nurs* **2**(9): 459–62

Pettigrew D (1989) Investing in mouth care. *Geriatr Nurs (Am J Care Aging)* **10**(1): 22–4

Poland JM (1987) Comparing moi-stir to lemon glycerine swabs. *Am J Nurs* **87**(4): 422–24

Price B (1990) *Body Image: Nursing concepts and care*. Prentice Hall, London: 215–16

Pyle MA, Massie M, Nelson S (1998) A pilot study on improving oral care in long-term care settings II: procedures and outcomes. *J Gerontol Nurs* **24**(10): 35–8

Ransier A, Epstein JB, Lunn R, Spinelli J (1995) A combined analysis of a toothbrush, foam brush, and a chlorhexidine-soaked foam brush in maintaining oral hygiene. *Cancer Nurs* **18**(5): 33–6

Rattenbury N, Mooney G, Bowen J (1999) Oral assessment and care for inpatients. *Nurs Times* **95**(49): 52–3

Regnard C, Allport S, Stephenson L (1997) ABC of palliative care. Mouth care, skin care, and lymphoedema. *Br Med J* **315**: 1002–5

Richardson A (1987) A process standard for oral care. *Nurs Times* **83**(32): 38–40

Rowe JA (2000) Accountability: a fundamental component of nursing practice. *Br J Nurs* **9**(9): 549–52

Royal College of Nursing (2000a) *Clinical Governance: How Nurses Can Get Involved*. RCN, London

Royal College of Nursing (2000b) *Rehabilitating Older People. The Role of the Nurse*. RCN, London

Ryan S (1996) Dry mouth misery. *Practice Nurse* **11**(3): 183–5

Ryrie I, Edwards M (1999) Assessment and planning for older people. In: Redfern SJ, Ross FM, eds. *Nursing Older People*. 3rd edn. Churchill Livingstone, London: 164–79

Shay K, Ship JA (1995) The importance of oral health in the older patient. *J Am Geriatr Soc* **43**(12): 1414–22

Shepherd G, Page C, Sammon P (1987) The mouth trap. *Nurs Times* **83**(19): 24–7

Ship JA (1999) The oral cavity. In: Hazzard WR, Blass JP, Ettinger WH, Halter JB, Ouslander JG, eds. *Principles of Geriatric Medicine and Gerontology*. 4th edn. McGraw-Hill, New York: 591–602

Simons D, Kidd EAM, Beighton D (1999) Oral health of elderly occupants in residential homes. *Lancet* **353**: 1761

Soames JV, Southam JC (1998) *Oral Pathology*. 3rd edn. Oxford University Press, Oxford

Speedie G (1983) Nursology of mouth care: preventing, comforting and seeking activities related to mouth care. *J Adv Nurs* **8**: 33–40

Steele JG (1996) Ageing in perspective. In: Murray JJ, ed. *Prevention of Oral Disease*. 3rd edn. Oxford University Press, Oxford: 189–99

Steele JG, Walls AWG (1997) Strategies to improve the quality of oral health care for frail and dependent older people. *Qual Health Care* **6**(3): 165–9

Sweeney MP, Shaw A, Yip B, Bagg J (1995) Oral health in elderly patients. *Br J Nurs* **4**(20): 1204–8

Sweeney P (1999) Oral health care for patients with mental illness. *J Nurs Care* **2**(1): 4–6

Sweeney P (1998a) Mouth care in nursing — part 1. Common oral conditions. *J Nurs Care* **1**(1): 4–7

Sweeney P (1998b) Mouth care in nursing — part 2. Oral mucosal infections. *J Nurs Care* **1**(2): 4–6

Sweeney P (1998c) Mouth care in nursing — part 3. Oral care for the dependent patient. *J Adv Nurs* **1**(3): 7–9

Thurgood G (1994) Nurse maintenance of oral hygiene. *Br J Nurs* **3**(7): 332–53

Tinker A (1997) *Older People in Modern Society*. 4th edn. Addison Wesley, London

Tombes MB, Gallucci B (1993) The effects of hydrogen peroxide rinses on the normal oral mucosa. *Nurs Res* **42**(6): 332–7

Torrance C (1990) Oral hygiene. *Surg Nurse* **3**(4): 16–20

Trenter Roth P, Creason NS (1986) Nurse administered oral hygiene: is there a scientific basis? *J Adv Nurs* **11**(3): 323–31

Turner G (1994) Oral care for patients who are terminally ill. *Nurs Standard* **8**(41): 49–54

Turner G (1996) Oral care. *Nurs Standard* **10**(28): 51–4

United Kingdom Central Council for Nursing, Midwifery and Health Visiting (1992) *Code of professional conduct for the nurse, midwife and health visitor*. UKCC, London

United Kingdom Central Council for Nursing, Midwifery and Health Visiting (1993) *Standards for Records and Record Keeping*. UKCC, London

United Kingdom Central Council for Nursing, Midwifery and Health Visiting (1996) *Guidelines for Professional Practice*. UKCC, London

Walls AWG (1996) Prevention in the ageing dentition. In: Murray JJ, ed. *Prevention of Oral Diseases*. 3rd edn. Oxford University Press, Oxford: chapter 13

Watson R (1989) Care of the mouth. *Nursing* **3**(44): 20–4

White R (2000) Nurse assessment of oral health: a review of practice and education. *Br J Nurs* **9**(5): 260–6

Whitmyer CC, Terezhalamy GT, Miller DL, Hujer ME (1998) Clinical evaluation of the efficacy and safety of an ultrasonic toothbrush system in an elderly patient population. *Geriatr Nurs* **18**(1): 29–33

Whitton C (1994) Symptoms that offer personal insight. Depression in elderly people. *Prof Nurse* **9**(4): 248–52

Wilkinson G, Miers M (1999) *Power and Nursing Practice*. Macmillan, London

Xavier G (2000) The importance of mouth care in preventing infection. *Nurs Standard* **14**(18): 47–51

Bibliography

Hoad-Reddick G, Heath JR (1995) Identification of elderly in particular need: results of a survey undertaken in residential homes in the Manchester area. *J Dentistry* **23**(5): 273–9

Meissner JE (1980) A simple guide for assessing oral health. *Nursing* **10**(4): 24–5

Pyle MA, Massie M, Nelson S (1998) A pilot study on improving oral care in long-term care settings. Part 1: oral health assessment. *J Gerontol Nurs* **24**(10): 31–4

Schweiger JL, Lang JW, Schweiger JW (1980) Oral assessment: how to do it. *Am J Nurs* **80**: 654–61

3

An exercise in the implementation of an oral hygiene protocol

Joan Curzio, Maggie McCowan

In 1997, the then Victoria Infirmary NHS Trust established a nursing research and practice development committee (NRPDC) to implement evidence-based practice in nursing care in response to its nursing strategy for 1998–2000. A survey of nursing projects was undertaken in 1996 and repeated in the spring of 1998. Initially, 107 projects were identified which included fifty-eight reviews of the literature. In 1998, ninety-five projects were identified with forty-two reviews of literature. The number of research projects being undertaken by nurses in the trust increased from four to fifteen and the number of audits increased from nine to forty-five. The NRPDC established a link nurse system to assist in developing practice at ward level and they have been offering a series of educational seminars. Oral hygiene was the first topic tackled trustwide, with a mouth care standard developed and staff knowledge subsequently surveyed six months after it was put into practice. Results demonstrated a good level of knowledge for general oral hygiene among trained and untrained staff. However, specialist oral care and care of stomatitis require some further updating. This survey has identified the increasing sophistication of the projects being undertaken by the nursing staff across the trust and the support they are receiving. This arrangement has provided the opportunity to demonstrate the impact of having a senior researcher available for advice at trust level. The NRPDC can improve the quality of evidence-based care delivered within the trust and it can provide a model for the implementation of evidence-based practice.

Evidence-based practice uses clinical expertise and research results to make decisions about the care of individual patients. With the advent of clinical governance and the corporate accountability for clinical practice, evidence-based practice is the means whereby clinical staff can account for their care. The gap between research and practice is well recognised. A number of studies have attempted to identify the barriers to research utilisation in nursing. These barriers include the lack of: time to implement new ideas; access to research facilities and skill to use them; critical appraisal skills; and organisational support for research (Foundation of Nursing Studies, 1996; Walsh, 1997; Dunn *et al*, 1998; le May *et al*, 1998; Newman *et al*, 1998).

From these and a number of similar studies within other professional groups, ways have been suggested to overcome such barriers (Burns and Grove, 1997; Grol, 1997; Jack and Oldham, 1997; Dunning *et al*, 1998). There have also been studies which have tested some of these methodologies (Kitson *et al*, 1996; Camiah, 1997; Pankhurst and Zainal, 1998) and an overall review (NHS Centre for Reviews and Dissemination, 1999).

There still remains a need to develop and evaluate further innovative methods to improve the flow of research-based knowledge through healthcare organisations and to individual practitioners. This is a report of the impact of a national research unit based in an acute trust working in conjunction with the local nursing research and practice development committee (NRPDC) to improve getting evidence into practice.

Background

The Nursing Research Initiative for Scotland (NRIS) is a funded research unit with a research and development remit within the Chief Scientist Office (CSO) that promotes, supports, participates in and develops research into multidisciplinary direct patient care. It is one of seven research units funded by the CSO, but the only one with a specific development remit and a clinical base within an acute trust. The NRPDC at the Victoria Infirmary NHS Trust, Glasgow, was formed in 1997 to support the implementation of the trust's recently formulated 'Nursing strategy'. Membership was drawn from across the trust and included: clinical managers, clinical nurse specialists, ward staff, midwives (while the maternity unit was still in existence), clinical audit and Scottish Intercollegiate Guideline Network (SIGN) implementation staff, and a representative from the NRIS whose clinical base is at the Victoria.

Methods

A case study approach (Simpson *et al*, 1997) was utilised to facilitate the evaluation of the joint workings of the committee and the NRIS in the trust. A number of steps were taken to set up organisational mechanisms and staff development opportunities (*Table 3.1*). These included establishing a network of link nurses whereby a member of staff from each unit agreed to be a 'link' with the committee for the cascade of information and to act as a local 'change agent'. Each trust member of the committee was assigned a group of link nurses.

Evaluation of the outcomes of this collaboration was carried out from several perspectives. A survey of nursing projects was conducted in 1996 before the inauguration of the committee and the setting up of the NRIS clinical base. A similar survey was completed in spring 1998. Results were tabulated, compared and graphed. In addition, general contacts with the NRIS were logged during the first fourteen months of operation and a similar period ending in 1998. These contacts were compared, including the types of staff seeking assistance and the reasons for consultation.

Table 3.1: Organisational mechanisms and staff development opportunities through the nursing research and practice development committee (NRPDC)

Individual members of staff or the committee identifies topic/perceived problem, actual problem, or review of practice	
Problems, topics and practices identified and committee's actions	⌘ Agrees to focus on issue
	⌘ Establishes current practice using link nurses and/or questionnaire
	⌘ Establishes evidence-based practice from the literature
	⌘ Identifies training needs between current practices and evidence-based practice
	⌘ Provides training, educational materials, or seminars
	⌘ Disseminates information via link nurses/seminars
	⌘ Evaluates, reports and disseminates results
Representation on trust committees	⌘ Director of nursing services and senior nurse group
	⌘ Guideline implementation group
	⌘ Clinical effectiveness committee
	⌘ Journal club
	⌘ Procedure committee
	⌘ Standards and audit committee
	⌘ Trust research and development group policy committee
Role of link nurses	⌘ One identified from each ward
	⌘ Each linked with a NRPDC member
	⌘ Encourage to attend seminars (see *Table 3.2*)

Oral hygiene was the first clinical topic to be targeted by the NRPDC. The evidence was reviewed (Buglass, 1995; Holmes, 1996; Mallet and Bailey, 1996; Sweeney, 1996). The current practice was assessed through a survey of current protocols in use across the trust, and trust-wide oral hygiene protocols were developed and finalised with the committee and link nurses (*Figure 3.1*). A survey of the oral hygiene knowledge of a random stratified sample of trained and untrained nursing staff was carried out six months after the introduction of the oral hygiene protocols.

Data were analysed and graphed using Microsoft Excel Version 7 for Windows 95. Statistical testing was undertaken using MINITAB version 11.2.

Oral hygiene protocols

Dentate patients (natural teeth)

- Natural teeth should be cleaned with fluoridated toothpaste after every meal, at least twice daily
- Partial dentures must be taken out and cleaned separately
- All patients must have their own toothbrush
- A dental hygienist or dentist should provide professional instruction and advice on oral hygiene for those with complex dental work, eg.bridges

- If patients are too unwell for normal oral methods seek professional dental advice
- Consider use of chlorhexidine mouthwash or spray (eg. Corsodyl®) for additional plaque control

> Many dependent patients cannot clean their own teeth and rely on nurses or other carers to provide oral hygiene measures

Edentulous patients (no natural teeth)

- All dentures should be marked with the patient's name (eg. 'Identure' Denture Marking System, Geri incorporated)
- Dentures should be left out of the mouth at night and soaked in a suitable cleansing solution — dilute sodium hypochlorite solution (eg. 1 part Milton 1% to 80 parts of water) for plastic dentures or chlorhexidine solution (eg. Corsodyl® 0.2%wv) for dentures with any metal parts. Rinse thoroughly before replacing in mouth
- Remember to check that the lining of the mouth is clean. If necessary, clean the oral mucosa with gauze or foam sticks moistened with water
- Dentures should be checked for cracks, sharp edges and missing teeth. Seek dental advice if necessary

> ### Denture hygiene
>
> - Dentures should be brushed at least once daily over a sink of water
> - Use of a personal toothbrush and running water are adequate for physical cleaning of dentures
> - Dentures should be rinsed thoroughly after meals
> - Dentures should be left out of the mouth at night

Prevention and treatment of staphylococcal mucositis

- Staphylococcal mucositis is a preventable condition. The key to prevention is regular oral hygiene (four times daily) provided by carers
- Treatment of established staphyloccal mucositis is by intensive oral lavage carried out three hourly. In selected cases flucloxacillin may be prescribed by medical staff but is not a substitute for oral hygiene
- To gain access to the mouth, dry cracked lips should be gently cleaned and moistened. The mucus crust inside the mouth should be softened and gently removed with a moistened gauze. If this results in bleeding, the cleaning can be completed by wiping with a gauze soaked in chlorhexidine (Corsodyl® 0.2%wv)
- Natural teeth may be brushed gently with chlorhexidine mouthwash. Never use toothpaste for these patients

> - Staphylococcal mucositis is a very distressing infection of the oral mucosa which may occur in patients with nasogastric or PEG tubes, those on IV fluids or unconscious patients who mouth-breath
> - Patients present with dry, crusted lips which may bleed. Inside the mouth a dry mucus crust can develop over all surfaces, especially the hard palate and tongue. When removed, this reveals a bleeding base

Remember
These patients represent
a serious aspiration risk

Figure 3.1: Oral hygiene protocols (Victoria Infirmary NHS Trust). PEG = percutaneous endoscopic gastrostomy; IV = intravenous

Joan Curzio, Maggie McCowan

Results

In total, twenty-eight nurses agreed to participate in the link nurse programme and five seminars were conducted from March 1997 to December 1998. The dates and educational topics covered during the seminars are listed in *Table 3.2*. Seminars also afforded the opportunity for the link nurses to participate in the clinical projects through discussion of results, protocols and consideration of future projects.

Table 3.2: Research and practice development link nurse seminars — educational component

March 1997	Presentation skills
June 1997	Basic statistical analysis
November 1997	None — only project work discussed
March 1998	How to conduct a search
November 1998	Integrated care pathways

A comparison of the outcomes of the 1996 and 1998 project surveys is shown in *Figure 3.2*. In 1996, 107 projects were identified and ninety-five projects were identified in 1998. Despite this slight reduction in total number of projects, there was an increase in the level of complexity of projects undertaken with fewer literature reviews being done in isolation. In 1996, fifty-eight reviews were carried out and only forty-two in 1998, but of these, twenty-four were done to support other categories of research and development (R&D) activity. There was a significant increase by Chi-square analysis in the number of research (P<0.01, $c2=6.971$, df=1) and audit (P<0.001, $c2=35.116$, df=1) projects reported. Overall, 48% reported receiving help from the NRIS in 1998 which included 93% of the research projects and 38% of the audit projects.

The general contacts with NRIS increased by 29% from 157 to 203 (*Figure 3.3*). There was a significant increase by Chi-square analysis in the proportion of staff nurses contacting the NRIS for assistance (P<0.01, $c2=7.394$, df=1). A total of 116 replies were received from the stratified random sample of 250 staff surveyed regarding their knowledge of oral hygiene.

The results indicated that staff knowledge of general oral hygiene and the treatment/prevention of Staphylococcal mucositis is good with 75% of the sample answering questions in this section accurately. However, specialist oral hygiene knowledge could be improved, eg. less than 50% of auxiliaries were able to identify accurately the proper techniques.

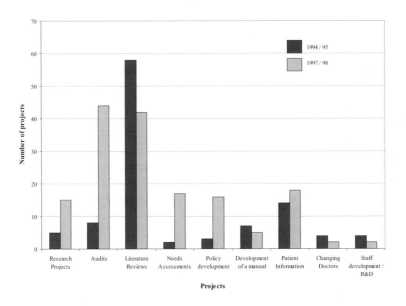

Figure 3.2: Projects surveyed 1996 and 1998. R&D = research and development

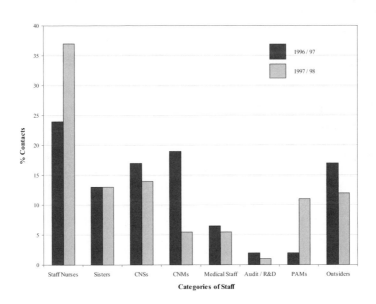

Figure 3.3: Contacts between staff at the Victoria Infirmary NHS Trust and the Nursing Research Initiative for Scotland. PAMs = professions allied to medicine; CNS = clinical nurse specialists; CNMs = clinical nurse managers; R&D = research and development

Discussion

A recent *Effective Health Care Bulletin* published by the NHS Centre for Reviews and Dissemination at the University of York (NHS Centre for Reviews and Dissemination, 1999) stresses that there appears to be no 'quick fix' for getting evidence into practice. Multifaceted interventions have been shown to be most effective, but in terms of changing professional behaviours, no intervention is effective under all circumstances. It would, therefore, seem that the general increase in research awareness activities presented and supported by NRIS and the NRPDC within the trust has created a fertile area for the implementation of research-based practice.

The educational seminars promoted the discussion of research findings in relationship to the nursing research and practice development agenda. Camiah (1997) has shown that the increasing confidence of the nursing staff when supported by a senior researcher has produced lively interactive debate and local consensus on the prioritised areas for practice development.

The structure of the NRPDC ensured that research into practice would be on the agenda at every managerial level. Interaction between other key committees was also assured with cross membership. One other aspect of the success of this venture was that the nurses felt ownership of the research was being implemented because it was relevant to their practice. The pertinent selection of the practice development priorities were decided by nursing staff who were aware of the strategy for the particular trust and the priorities of the NRIS working within an acute trust. Lack of supportive organisation and structures and lack of access to research expertise have previously been identified as barriers (le May *et al*, 1998).

This collaboration has attempted to address a number of the barriers to research and evidence-based practice. Easy access to bibliographic databases, education on how to search and critique the literature to establish mechanisms for identifying and tackling local clinical problems have all been addressed. There has been a demonstratively significant increase in the number of research and audit projects undertaken in the trust by nursing staff. The NRIS clinical base has demonstrated an involvement in many of these projects and participated directly in the NRPDC work as well.

Conclusions

This work indicates that the uptake of research findings and general involvement in research can be improved with the support of a national research unit on site and a committed local research and practice development committee.

The Nursing Research Initiative for Scotland is a chief scientist office (CSO) funded research unit and the views expressed are those of the authors and not necessarily those of the funded body.

Key points

⌘ Nursing staff are undertaking sophisticated projects and receive much support for their work.

⌘ It is important to have a senior researcher available for advice.

⌘ Having representation from all managerial levels facilitates implementation of evidence-based practice.

⌘ Through the use of link nurses and seminars, a wide range of staff have been able to participate in developing evidence-based practice.

⌘ When initiating wide changes, it is better to focus on common areas of nursing practice.

References

Buglass EA (1995) Oral hygiene. *Br J Nurs* **4**(9): 516–19

Burns N, Grove SK (1997) Utilization of research in nursing practice. In: *The Practice of Nursing Research: Conduct, Critique and Utilization*. 3rd edn. WB Saunders, London: 671–701

Camiah S (1997) Utilization of nursing research in practice and application strategies to raise research awareness among nurse practitioners: a model for success. *J Adv Nurs* **26**: 1193–202

Dunn V, Crichton N, Roe B, Seers K, Willians K (1998) Using research for practice: a UK experience of the BARRIERS Scale. *J Adv Nurs* **27**: 1203–10

Dunning M, Abi-Aad G, Gilbert D, Gillam S, Livett H (1998) *Turning Evidence into Everyday Practice: An Interim Report from the Pace Programme*. King's Fund, London

Foundation of Nursing Studies (1996) *Reflection for Action: An Exploration of National and Local Nursing Research Implementation Cultures; Barriers, Expectations and Achievements and Identifying Opportunities for the Future*. Foundation of Nursing Studies, London

Grol R (1997) Beliefs and evidence in changing clinical practice. *Br Med J* **315**: 418–21

Holmes S (1996) Nursing management of oral care in older patients. *Nurs Times* **92**(28): 37–9

Jack B, Oldham J (1997) Taking steps towards evidence-based practice: a model for implementation. *Nurse Researcher* **5**(1): 65–71

Kitson A, Ahmed LB, Harvey G, Seers K, Thompson DR (1996) From research to practice: one organizational model for promoting research-based practice. *J Adv Nurs* **23**: 430–40

le May A, Alexander C, Mulhall A (1998) Research utilization in nursing: barriers and opportunities. *J Clin Effectiveness* **3**(2): 59–63

Mallet J, Bailey C (1996) *The Royal Marsden NHS Trust: Annual of Clinical Nursing Procedures*. 4th edn. Blackwell Science, Bath

Newman M, Papadopoulos I, Sigsworth J (1998) Barriers to evidence-based practice. *Clin Effectiveness Nurs* **2**: 11–20

NHS Centre for Reviews and Dissemination (1999) *Effective Health Care Bulletin: Getting Evidence into Practice*. Royal Society of Medicine Press, London

Pankhurst FL, Zainal G (1998) Putting research into practice: overcoming the barriers. *Managing Clinical Nursing* **2**: 81–6

Simpson V, Curzio J, Gillespie A, McCowan M (1997) Evidence-based practice: a case study. *Nurs Times* (Research) **2**(6): 426–32

Sweeney P (1996) *Down in the mouth* (oral hygiene video). Glasgow University Media Department, Glasgow

Walsh M (1997) How nurses perceive barriers to research implementation. *Nurs Standard* **11**(29): 34–9

4

An audit of oral care practice and staff knowledge in hospital palliative care

L Lee, V White, J Ball, K Gill, L Smart, K McEwan, P Chilton, P Pickering

Mouth care is considered one of the most basic of nursing activities, and palliative care patients are especially vulnerable to oral problems (Macmillan Practice Development Unit, 1995). This chapter describes a project on developing oral care practice and staff knowledge, by nursing staff and Macmillan nurses at a hospital in central England. A baseline audit (audit I) was carried out to examine all aspects of current oral care practice and nursing knowledge, including assessment, implementation, prescribing and evaluation of care. Oral care guidelines and a programme of ward-based teaching were then introduced. Several months later a follow-up audit (audit II) was conducted. Results showed an improvement in all aspects of oral care and staff knowledge. Additional benefits of this process included improved professional relationships and the promotion of further audits in hospital palliative care. Recommendations include the need for further nursing research into oral care to build the evidence base further. Additionally, it is suggested that nurses must recognise their important and central role in improving this aspect of palliative care. Education and training is pivotal to this process.

Improved patient care is a long-term aim of government health policy in the UK, but the focus of change to deliver this aim varies from government to government. A range of recent documents (Department of Health [DoH], 1998, 1999, 2001; NHS Executive, 1999) have placed an emphasis on evaluation as a quality-control tool. Additionally, quality has been placed on the palliative care agenda by more specific documents (eg. National Council for Hospice and Specialist Palliative Care Services [NCHSPCS], 1997). Clinical audit is a vital part of this improvement process in palliative care and the wider healthcare services.

This chapter describes an audit project conducted by hospital nursing staff and the palliative care clinical nurse specialists (Macmillan nurses) in Newark Hospital, Nottinghamshire, UK, with the aim of improving oral care practice and nurse knowledge. The audit group was convened following a programme of palliative care education for the ward managers provided by the Macmillan team. At the end of this course, which lasted for six months, it was decided that guidelines for oral care were required to standardise and improve the oral care provided to palliative care patients in this general hospital. This chapter begins by reviewing the literature regarding staff knowledge and clinical practice of oral care. The audit methodology is then described and the results presented and discussed.

Literature review

Information regarding oral care was gathered from a previously-published literature review (Macmillan Practice Development Unit, 1995) and from a search conducted on the CINAHL database using the terms 'mouth care', 'oral care' and 'oral hygiene'.

Oral care problems appear to be commonplace for cancer and palliative care patients (Macmillan Practice Development Unit, 1995). The presence of oral problems often causes discomfort and may precipitate further complications (Ohrn *et al*, 2000), therefore mouth care needs to be performed thoroughly at all stages of the cancer journey in order to enhance the quality of patients' lives (Ohrn *et al*, 2000). The condition of a patient's mouth can also indicate the quality of his/her care and regular inspection of it should be regarded as a basic nursing duty.

From our limited search it appears that little research has been carried out on education about, and knowledge of, mouth care among nursing staff. Curzio and McGowan's (2000) study suggested that the basic level of oral hygiene knowledge among the trained and untrained staff in a Scottish hospital was good, although any specialist knowledge was lacking. However, less than 50% of untrained staff were able to identify the correct technique for oral care and only 5% of all nurses felt they had enough knowledge of mouth care (Curzio and McGowan, 2000). Ohrn *et al* (2000) have also acknowledged that further training is needed for nurses. This is not surprising when, in palliative care for example, few texts discuss oral care in any depth. Some authors mention oral care in just a few lines (eg. Twycross, 1995), while others only comment on it in regard to final phase care (eg. Doyle, 1994).

In order to provide good quality oral care, a full assessment of the patient's mouth and oral status is required (Krishnasamy, 1995). However, Freer (2000) found that assessment was often given a low priority due to heavy workloads. Although attempts to form an assessment tool have been made (Eilers *et al*, 1988; Jenkins, 1989; Freer, 2000), there is not yet a standard tool that is easy to use with the demands of the current healthcare climate (eg. lack of time), or that has been tested in palliative care. Although the literature suggests Eilers *et al*'s (1988) assessment tool and the categories included in it are appropriate for palliative care patients, replication studies are required.

Oral care should be part of every palliative care patient's ongoing care plan. However, the provision of good quality oral care is not always apparent in general health care (Adams, 1996) or palliative care (Mahaffey, 1997). Reasons given by nurses for poor mouth care are lack of time (Boyle, 1992) and lack of knowledge (Ohrn *et al*, 2000). In addition, the frequency with which mouth care is provided may vary from once every shift, to only if the patient requests it (Krishnasamy, 1995). Despite regularity being regarded as vital, it is often dependent on the intention of the mouth care procedure and requires an individual approach; for example, if the aim is to reduce oral complications and promote comfort then two-hourly mouth care is required (Macmillan Practice Development Unit, 1995).

Additionally, the tools used in mouth care have been criticised for being used ritualistically (Moore, 1995), eg. nurses have often preferred to use foam sticks rather than a toothbrush as the primary tool for providing oral care (Peate, 1993) even though literature suggests that they are ineffective at cleaning tooth surfaces (Crosby, 1989). This preference for foam sticks could reflect nurses' lack of training on appropriate oral care equipment. However, foam sticks may be chosen because they are quicker to use, and therefore preferred by nurses given their time constraints and heavy workloads. Evidence and further research is required about patients' perceptions of the use of the differing oral care tools.

From the relative lack of literature and research evidence available, it seems that nurses cannot be held fully responsible for poor oral care, which is a result of outdated, unstandardised, ritualistic practices (Krishnasamy, 1995; Moore, 1995; Mahaffey, 1997). Nevertheless, oral care is a core aspect of nursing care and nurses must therefore consider undertaking further research, audits and quality initiatives to enhance the evidence base. This need for standardisation and improvement in oral care and nursing knowledge provided the impetus for the following audit.

Developing the guidelines

The process of developing oral care guidelines for the Central Nottingham Healthcare Trust began in 1998. The guidelines were based on a consensus of opinion from the audit team and derived from the evidence-based literature then available. They were peer reviewed within the trust, and ratified by the trust's policies and procedures group.

The scientific merit of guidelines is dependent on the availability and quality of literature used (Grimshaw and Russell, 1993). Difficulties are therefore apparent in specialties such as palliative care where research is not always available (Corner, 1996). The comprehensive review of the oral care literature from the Macmillan Practice Development Unit (1995) was used as a basis for our guidelines. The guidelines included information on their anticipated benefits, potential client group, measurable outcomes, assessment of oral care, treatment principles for basic oral care, appropriate tools and agents, and various management options for specific oral care problems, eg. dry mouth (*Box 4.1*).

The guidelines were appraised using a clinical guideline assessment

---

Box 4.1: Management options for patients with dry mouths

❖ Stop causative drug if possible and relevant

❖ Exclude oral infection, eg. oral thrush

❖ Encourage intake of drinks, crushed ice, boiled sweets

❖ If acceptable patient should chew pieces of pineapple chunks

❖ If acceptable patient should chew gum to stimulate saliva

❖ Consider saliva substitutes

❖ Keep lips moist

Source: Extract from guidelines

---

instrument developed by a group of UK medical and dentistry schools (Cluzeau *et al*, 1997). This instrument contains thirty-seven questions addressing different aspects of guideline development, including rigour, context, content and application. These issues are considered to ensure the validity of any guidelines (Grimshaw and Russell, 1993).

Audits of oral care practice and knowledge

Before dissemination of the guidelines in late 1998, an audit (audit I) was undertaken to identify the standards of oral care practice and staff knowledge at that time. The audit team consisted of two Macmillan nurses, two ward managers and four staff nurses from one surgical and two medical wards in the hospital. This was the same team that had developed the oral care guidelines.

Two tools were used in this process. The first was a standardised oral care practice questionnaire developed by the audit team, based on the aspects of care included in the guidelines. It covered the physical assessment of the patient's oral care status, equipment used, medication prescribed, advice given to patients and nursing documentation completed. Three nurses from the audit team aimed to complete a maximum of ten randomly selected practice questionnaires for patients on each of three (one surgical and two medical) wards (ie. n=30). These patients were randomised by the audit team choosing every third patient on the ward. Information was gathered from the patients themselves, as well as their notes.

The second tool was a questionnaire used to assess the current status of knowledge of all hospital staff, and its content again reflected the guidelines. These tools were similar for both trained and untrained members of staff and covered aspects of oral care practice. For trained nurses questions on medication were also included. All nursing staff on the three wards were given this questionnaire, which was returned anonymously. The Macmillan nurses collated the results.

Once the baseline standard of care and knowledge had been identified, the guidelines were disseminated through ward-based education. Teaching sessions, which lasted for approximately thirty minutes, were made available to all trained and untrained nurses, as well as student nurses on placement. The focus of the sessions was based on the weaknesses and gaps in knowledge identified from audit I as well as the focus of the guidelines, such as assessment, mouth care tools and agents, patient advice, documentation and specific oral care problems. The teaching took place towards the end of 1999 and was undertaken by the ward members of the audit team. The teaching incorporated a number of formal sessions on each ward and a note was made of which members had attended. The sessions continued until all nursing staff had been to a teaching session. In addition, a mouth care information package was devised by one of the surgical nurses and each clinical area had access to a copy of this.

Finally, in 2000, after a consolidation period of three months, the final phase of the study was undertaken. The audit process of assessing the oral care knowledge of all members of staff and practice based on the assessment of the care of thirty patients was repeated (audit II). The process was identical to audit I and once the Macmillan team had collated the results, they were compared with those of audit I to identify any changes in knowledge and practice. It is not known whether there were any changes in staff members employed by the hospital between the implementation of audits I and II, although the audit team believe that any changes in staff members would have been minimal and therefore unlikely to greatly influence the audit results.

Audit results

In audit I only seventeen oral care practice questionnaires (56%) were completed. The oral care knowledge questionnaires had a 58% response rate for trained staff and a 45% response rate for untrained staff. In audit II, twenty-seven practice questionnaires (90%) were completed, and there was a 50% response rate for trained staff, and 61% for untrained staff, on the knowledge questionnaires. These response rates for audit I were disappointing, despite calls for more questionnaires to be completed and returned. Available time and winter pressures of increased workloads during audit I may have made the return of questionnaires difficult.

Oral care practice

The quality of oral care practice was separated into four categories by looking at the overall standard of assessment, documentation and implementation of oral care and comparing the results with the recommendations in the guidelines (*Table 4.1*). Results indicate that the number of overall poor oral care practice audits were reduced in audit II from 7% to 4% and the number of good overall oral care practice audits increased from 20% to 56%. Other categories also showed movement towards favourable results. These results suggest that the nurse is in a prime position to bring about improvements in patients' oral care.

Audit I identified that 77% of patients had oral care problems potentially requiring medication. However, only 20% of these patients actually had medication prescribed, and 10% of these prescriptions were inappropriate; for example, nystatin was prescribed when no oral thrush was identified. This audit did not identify why 57% of patients were not prescribed anything. Prescribing for oral care showed improvements in audit II: results identified that 71% of patients had oral care problems requiring medication, and 71% of these patients had oral care medication prescribed, none of which were inappropriate. Appropriately prescribed medication included nystatin, fluconazole, vitamin C and certain mouthwashes.

Table 4.1: Overall standard of oral care practice among trained staff (%)

Standard of oral care practice	Audit I (n=17)	Audit II (n=27)
No good assessment, documentation or implementation of oral care	7	4
Good assessment of oral care, poor documentation and implementation	40	32
Good assessment and documentation but poor implementation of oral care	33	8
Good assessment, documentation and implementation of oral care	20	56

The advice that staff gave to patients was also audited, based on the patient's recollection of this. In audit I, 30% of patients said they had been given advice regarding timing of mouth care, use of foam sticks, lip salve and sweets. In audit II, 46% of patients said they or their relatives had been given advice which extended to include the use of pineapple, ice, fizzy drinks, and use of prescribed products such as vitamin C. Advice given to patients and their carers is recognised as being pivotal in reducing further problems (Bersani and Carl, 1983) as continual mouth care undertaken by patients or carers themselves can prevent oral complications. Indeed, simple measures are often enough to promote a clean moist mouth and prevent problems occurring.

Use of equipment or products for oral care was audited (*Table 4.2*) and changes in the use of certain oral care tools and products were found between audits. It is important to note that during the ward managers' educational programme in 1997, the use of lemon and glycerine moist sticks was identified as poor practice (Cheater, 1985). The recorded use of these products in audit I was only 8%, possibly due to the ward manager's awareness of this. The audit team believe the use of these lemon and glycerine sticks was much higher before the educational programme. Although figures are not available, pharmacy stock usage suggests this. In audit II this figure was reduced to 0%, in line with the guidelines.

Audit II also identified an increase in the use of toothpaste and toothbrushes, complying with evidence suggesting that this is best practice where possible, even in those patients unable to carry out independent mouth care (Bersani and Carl, 1983; Krishnasamy, 1995). It has been proposed that toothpaste, which contains fluoride, lowers the surface tension on the teeth, which in turn facilitates the loosening of debris from the teeth (Macmillan Practice Development Unit, 1995).

The increased use of pineapple from 0% in audit I to 21% in audit II is of importance. Despite the lack of conclusive evidence to support its value, pineapple is considered to cleanse and promote saliva production in a dry mouth (Krishnasamy, 1995), although further research is needed.

Finally, the nurses' documentation of oral care practice were audited (*Table 4.3*). Results showed that on the whole the documentation of oral care had improved. This moderate increase could indicate an improved appreciation and awareness of continuous oral care. However, a further improvement in all documentation was identified as a goal for the future by the audit team.

Table 4.2: Mouth care equipment and products used by trained staff (%)

Mouth care equipment/products used	Audit I (*n*=17)	Audit II (*n*=27)
Toothbrush	46	79
Toothpaste	38	71
Foam sticks	69	50
Mouthwash	77	63
Denture pot	23	46
Lip vaseline	8	13
Lemon/glycerine sticks	8	0
Ice	0	4
Pineapple	0	21

Table 4.3: Nurses' documentation of oral care practice (%)

Oral care documentation	Audit I (*n*=17)	Audit II (*n*=27)
Oral assessment completed on admission on the activities of daily living form	69	79
Problem documented in patient's notes	39	63
Written evaluation of oral care provided	31	46
Oral care documented as a care plan	46	56

Oral care knowledge

The results of the knowledge questionnaires showed a general increase in knowledge for all groups of staff after the ward training (*Tables 4.4* and *4.5*). This highlights the importance of education provision within any audit implementation process (Higginson *et al*, 1996) and oral care practice.

Untrained staff had the greatest increase in knowledge (*Table 4.4*) with favourable changes in both the lowest and highest scores. Knowledge increased specifically on practical aspects of oral care, eg. tools or products used and patient advice. The trained staff (*Table 4.5*) also displayed similar favourable changes in the lowest and highest scores. Knowledge among the trained staff increased positively on all aspects of oral care from documentation and assessment to implementation and medication.

Table 4.4: Oral care knowledge for untrained staff

Knowledge scores	Audit I (n=14)	Audit II (n=19)
Mean score (out of 20)	8(40%)	13(65%)
Lowest score (out of 20)	2(10%)	9(45%)
Highest score (out of 20)	14(70%)	18(90%)

Table 4.5: Oral care knowledge for trained staff

Knowledge scores	Audit I (n=35)	Audit II (n=30)
Mean score (out of 24)	14(58%)	18(75%)
Lowest score (out of 24)	7(29%)	12(50%)
Highest score (out of 24)	23(96%)	24(100%)

Discussion

The audit and work involved resulted in many positive outcomes. The study strengthened professional relationships between the Macmillan team and ward staff, resulting in a change in oral care practice, generating learning for the group on audit procedures, and acknowledging good organisational support. It also highlighted the commitment and concerted efforts of everyone to improve the quality of hospital palliative care.

A considerable factor in this study's success was that the staff working on the wards initiated, developed and undertook the guidelines and audit. Indeed, 'ownership' of any changes in practice maximises commitment (McPhail, 1997). The successful implementation of any guidelines or audits should include the factors outlined in *Box 4.2*.

> **Box 4.2: Ways to implement successfully guidelines or audits**
>
> ❖ Clear communication
> ❖ Bottom-up approach
> ❖ Time dedicated to professional training
> ❖ Support from local audit department
> ❖ Making use of existing knowledge and specialists
> ❖ A managed process

Audit limitations

Although the results illustrate improved clinical practice and knowledge of oral care, the audit has a number of limitations. Despite the audit tools being specifically designed for this study, they were not extensively tested for their reliability and validity. However, the tools were tested and revised in a pilot phase and the information produced was considered acceptable to the members of the working group and audit department. Additionally, the knowledge audit tools tested actual oral care practice rather than self-ratings of the perceived knowledge increase; this is deemed more reliable (Ohrn *et al*, 2000).

Unfortunately, with the exception of one group, the response rates from the knowledge questionnaires were under 60%. Low response rates (those below 60%) are a recognised disadvantage of using self-responding questionnaires (Polit and Hungler, 2000). However, within an audit context, questionnaires are considered more conducive to repetition and dispersion than face-to-face interviews (Jacoby *et al*, 1999).

Change is a complex process. Indeed, there has been scepticism as to the effect of audit and feedback in showing any change in clinical practice (Richardson, 1999) and palliative care (Higginson *et al*, 1996). However, a number of audits undertaken in palliative care contexts have encouraged or shown changes in practice (Baldry and Balmer, 2000; Ling, 2000). Change and favourable results depend on many factors including the people involved, peer influence, organisational issues, administrative procedures, communication, difficulties encountered and the education provided (McPhail, 1997). Difficulties encountered within this audit included professional demands and pressures, unmet deadlines, the need for considerable investment of time and energy from the entire group and the need to maintain motivation over the two years the project took to complete.

Conclusion

The audit results acknowledge the positive effect of the process on both staff knowledge and clinical oral care, thereby helping to improve this aspect of palliative care in the hospital setting. All members of the audit team concluded that the procedures adopted were challenging but rewarding. Recommendations for further research and for nurses to acknowledge their central role in improving oral care practice have been made. Additionally, interest was spurred to develop further guidelines and audits on other issues relevant to palliative care, both in this group and a wider multiprofessional arena. Initiatives discussed for the future include guidelines for constipation and breaking bad news.

We would like to thank all the patients and staff who made this audit possible. In particular we would like to thank the hospital managers who supported the time taken by all hospital staff involved, to undertake this project.

Key points

⌘ Oral care should be part of the palliative care plan.

⌘ Many patients in palliative care have oral care problems that require medication. However, medication is often either inappropriate or under-dispensed.

⌘ An audit cycle was effective in bringing about an increase in the use of toothpaste and toothbrushes, pineapple for cleansing and saliva production, and, improved documentation.

References

Adams R (1996) Qualified nurses lack adequate knowledge related to oral health resulting in inadequate oral care of patients on medical wards. *J Adv Nurs* **24**: 552–60

Baldry C, Balmer S (2000) An audit of out of hours advice services provided by hospice staff. *Int J Palliat Nurs* **6**(7): 352–9

Bersani G, Carl W (1983) Oral care for cancer patients. *Am J Nurs* **83**(4): 533–6

Boyle S (1992) Assessing mouth care. *Nurs Times* **88**: 44–6

Cheater F (1985) Xerostomia in malignant disease. *Nurs Mirror* **161**: 3

Cluzeau F, Littlejohns P, Grimshaw J, Feder G (1997) *Appraisal Instrument for Clinical Guidelines*. St George's Hospital Medical School, London

Corner J (1996) Is there a research paradigm for palliative care? *Palliat Med* 10: 201–8

Crosby C (1989) Method in mouth care. *Nurs Times* **76**: 48–51

Curzio J, McGowan M (2000) Getting research into practice: developing oral hygiene standards. *Br J Nurs* **9**(7): 434–8

Department of Health (1998) *A First Class Service:Quality in the New NHS*. DoH, London

Department of Health (1999) *Making a Difference: Strengthening the Nursing, Midwifery and Health Visiting Contribution to Health and Healthcare*. DoH, London

Department of Health (2001) *The Essence of Care: Patient Focused Benchmarking for Health Care Practitioners*. DoH, London

Doyle D (1994) *Domiciliary Palliative Care: A Guide for the Primary Health Care Team*. Oxford University Press, Oxford

Eilers J, Bergen A, Peterson M (1988) Development, testing and application of the oral assessment guide. *Oncol Nurs Forum* **15**: 325–30

Freer SK (2000) Use of an oral assessment tool to improve practice. *Prof Nurse* **15**(10): 635–7

Grimshaw J, Russell I (1993) Achieving health gain through clinical guidelines I: developing scientifically valid guidelines. *Qual Health Care* **2**: 243–8

Higginson IJ, Hearn J, Webb D (1996) Audit in palliative care: does practice change? *Eur J Cancer Care* **5**: 233–6

Jacoby A, Le Couturier J, Bradshaw C, Lovel T, Eccles M (1999) Feasibilty of using a postal questionnaire to examine carer satisfaction with palliative care: a methodological assessment. *Palliat Med* **13**(4): 275–84

Jenkins DA (1989) Oral care in ICU: an important nursing role. *Nurs Standard* **4**(7): 24–8

Krishnasamy M (1995) Oral care problems in advanced cancer. *Eur J Cancer Care* **4**: 173–7

Ling J (2000) Audit in practice: the referral of dying patients to palliative care. *Int J Palliat Nurs* **6**(8): 375–9

Macmillan Practice Development Unit (1995) *Managing Oral Care Problems throughout the Cancer Illness Trajectory*. Macmillan Practice Development Unit, London

Mahaffey W (1997) Research based mouth care in palliative care patients in the community setting. *Int J Palliat Nurs* **3**(6): 330–3

McPhail G (1997) The management of change: an essential skill for nursing in the 1990s. *J Nurs Manag* **5**(4): 199–205

Moore J (1995) Assessment of nurse administered oral hygiene. *Nurs Times* **91**(9): 40–1

National Council for Hospice and Specialist Palliative Care Services (1997) *Making Palliative Care Better: Quality Improvements, Multiprofessional Audit and Standards.* Occasional paper 12. NCHSPCS, London

NHS Executive (1999) *Clinical Governance: Quality in the New NHS.* DoH, London

Ohrn K, Wahlin Y, Sjoden P (2000) Oral care in cancer nursing. *Eur J Cancer Care* **9**(1): 22–9

Peate I (1993) Nurse administered oral hygiene in the hospitalised patient. *Br J Nurs* **2**(9): 459–62

Polit DF, Hungler BP (2000) *Nursing Research: Principles and Methods.* Lippincott, London

Ralph D (2000) Mouth piece. *Nurs Standard* **14**(35): 26

Richardson R (1999) Implementing evidenced based practice. *Prof Nurse* **15**(2): 101–4

Twycross R (1995) *Introducing Palliative Care.* Radcliffe Medical Press, Oxford

5

Mouth care in cancer nursing: using the audit cycle to change practice

Amanda Honnor, Annie Law

Patients with cancer face an assault on oral health from their disease and accompanying treatment options and are vulnerable to developing oral problems; therefore, the maintenance of oral health is particularly important. A study was carried out in one oncology unit within a large teaching hospital to measure the extent of oral problems in cancer patients, current mouth care practices, and staff knowledge. The findings showed that oral problems were common, but were: (1) underreported by patients, (2) underdiagnosed by doctors and nurses, (3) inadequately treated, and (4) inadequately documented. Nursing staff were found to have knowledge deficits. Changes to practice as a result of these findings included the development and implementation of an oral assessment tool and the development of oral care guidelines; additionally, patient information leaflets and posters were produced and a staff education programme was introduced. A further audit found that there had been significant improvements in the diagnosis and treatment of oral problems and increased reporting of previously ignored problems by patients.

Oral problems were regularly observed by the authors in patients within the oncology unit of a large teaching hospital within the East Midlands. The purpose of this study was to ascertain the extent of these problems and to determine whether the care and treatment being delivered was evidence based and if the people delivering mouth care had sufficient related knowledge. Oral hygiene currently has a high profile as one of the eight clinical benchmarks proposed as part of the nursing strategy (Department of Health [DoH], 1999a) and in *The Essence of Care* document (DoH, 2001).

Search the evidence

A number of strategies were used to search the literature for identification of relevant studies. Electronic databases searched were Medline, CINAHL, British Nursing Index, and the Cochrane Database between 1975 and 2001. This search was carried out before developing the audit tool. This chapter is not intended to be a comprehensive review of mouth care, but aims to identify why cancer patients are particularly vulnerable to oral problems.

Why do cancer patients have oral problems?

Patients with cancer face an assault on oral health from their disease and accompanying treatment options and are vulnerable to oral problems; therefore, the maintenance of oral health is particularly important (Crosby, 1989; Poland, 1991; Porter, 1994). Within cancer care, complications associated with particular types of treatment can have devastating effects on the oral cavity. Many chemotherapy drugs such as methotrexate, 5-fluorouracil, cyclophosphamide, doxorubicin, and bleomycin are commonly associated with oral problems (Knox *et al*, 2000).

Chemotherapy has a two-stage effect on the mouth. Within four to seven days thinning and ulceration of the mucosa occurs. Nausea, vomiting, and general malaise, caused by the treatment, compound the problem by reducing food and fluid intake and allowing plaque and debris to accumulate on the teeth and mucosal surfaces (Crosby, 1989). This makes the mucosa an ineffective barrier to opportunistic infections (Driezen *et al*, 1982; Porter, 1994; Gibson *et al*, 1997). Within ten to sixteen days following initiation of each cycle of chemotherapy, myelosuppression can result in neutropenia and thrombo-cytopenia causing the mucosa to be further susceptible to infection and haemorrhage (Crosby, 1989).

Stomatitis is a common problem following certain chemotherapy treatments, resulting in pain, ulceration and possibly leading to haemorrhage and infection. Most documented oral infections in chemotherapy patients actually originate from their own microflora (Allbright, 1984). Severe mucositis can lead to ulceration and erosions which can cause such severe pain that therapy may need to be suspended as, by this time, the patient may be unable to eat and drink and could become severely nutritionally depleted (Coleman, 1995). Complications such as mucositis may also have far-reaching psychological effects in that halitosis may lead to avoidance between the patient and a loved one and dry and cracked lips may lead to difficulties in speaking and expressing affection. Mucositis is a major contributor to therapy-related morbidity and mortality (Trenter Roth *et al*, 1986; Berger and Eilers,1998).

The other modality of treatment which can have a devastating effect on the oral cavity is radiotherapy. The dose, fractionation, and treatment field determine damage to the mouth caused by radiation. Owing to the local effect on cellular replication, mucositis may occur. The salivary glands may be affected causing the saliva to be more viscous or even absent. This results in swallowing and taste disturbances, and affects the normal protective environment of the mouth, leaving the patient vulnerable to dental decay (Allbright, 1984).

There is evidence to suggest that systemic infection, originating in the mouth may lead to septicaemia, which is the primary cause of death in a significant number of cancer patients (McElroy, 1984; Crosby, 1989; Porter, 1994).

What the literature says about staff knowledge

One of the most basic nursing activities is mouth care (Macmillan Practice Development Unit, 1995) and it has been suggested that the state of a patient's mouth is a good indicator of the general standard of patient care, implying that if the patient's oral hygiene is poor the general standard of care is poor. Yet, frequently the task of administering mouth care is allocated to junior or auxiliary staff (Henderson, 1960; Crosby, 1989; Peate, 1993).

Nurses in the United Kingdom nurses receive inadequate training in oral health assessment and care (White, 2000). Oral care is rarely taught by experts in the field, and many nurse training establishments have oral care syllabus deficiencies. Students were found to have been recommended books which had insufficient information to provide an insight into oral care or dental disease (Longhurst, 1998). Recommendations were made with respect to an urgent need for the dental and nursing professions to liaise in order to remedy this situation (Barnett, 1991) and it was recommended that nurses who normally administer oral care should be taught by dental hygienists (Howarth, 1977; Lewis, 1984).

Adams (1996) undertook a study to ascertain the knowledge of oral care among qualified nurses working on medical wards and found that they lacked adequate knowledge. Similar findings were reported by Boyle (1992) who found that qualified nurses received little or no oral care instruction during their basic training. In a study by Lee *et al* (2001) gaps in nursing knowledge were clearly identified, but following the development and implementation of written guidelines, a significant improvement was noted.

There is evidence to suggest that nurses carry out oral care in a ritualistic way simply because that is the way it has always been done (Clarke, 1993; Hatton-Smith, 1994). Criticism from peers may be a factor in preventing nurses from implementing improvements in care, as they fear incurring the wrath of their colleagues (Hatton-Smith, 1994), or it may be due to confusion surrounding the choice of implement, cleansing agent, and frequency of oral care, resulting in nurses feeling uncertain as to what oral regimes they should follow (Gibson *et al*, 1997). Ohrn *et al* (2000) suggest that there has been little investigation into the obstacles to staff performing oral care, particularly relating to education and knowledge.

What the literature says about evidence-based mouth care

Before the 1970s, nursing did not possess any significant research base and could not be said to have a body of knowledge unique to itself (Walsh and Ford, 1989). The equipment used to carry out oral care is very important. There is strong evidence to suggest that the toothbrush is the most effective tool for oral care (Clarke, 1993; Moore, 1995; Pearson, 1996). However, in research carried out to investigate nurses' use of tools, Adams (1996) found that of the thirty-five nurses involved in her study, only ten mentioned the use of toothbrushes for mouth care, preferring foam swabs.

Many of the tools, other than toothbrushes and the various solutions used by nurses for mouth care, eg. sponges on sticks, lemon and glycerine swabs, forceps with gauze swabs are of unproven value and some are possibly harmful (Kite and Pearson, 1995; Bowsher *et al*, 1999). The effectiveness of the various solutions has been discussed in a recent article by Milligan *et al* (2001) and it is not within the scope of this chapter to repeat this information. However, they found that frequency of care and regular assessment of the oral cavity contributed to improvements in oral health as much as the use of any one solution alone and the evidence surrounding the use of tools was contradictory. Moore (1995) and Hatton-Smith (1994) maintain that despite research validating the need for good oral care, it is often a time-wasting ritual based not on evidence but on tradition.

The aim of our study was to evaluate current practice and implement any changes required to ensure oral care was clinically effective and evidence-based.

Clinical effectiveness

All healthcare professionals strive to provide clinically effective care. Clinical effectiveness is about doing the right thing in the right way and at the right time for the right patient (Royal College of Nursing [RCN], 1996). There are several key activities needed to support clinically effective practice:

- selecting a particular practice to question or examine
- searching for and critically appraising the literature and other sources for evidence of best practice
- auditing practice to confirm whether you are providing best practice
- changing practice to make improvements required (Rosenberg and Donald, 1995; White, 1997).

Clinical audit

The White Paper *Working for Patients* (DoH, 1989) raised the profile of audit, now recognised as an integral part of the work of all those involved in healthcare delivery (DoH, 1989). Continuous professional development should focus on the development needs of clinical audit and putting in place service improvements based on audit findings (DoH, 1999b). Clinical audit is a clinically led initiative, which seeks to improve the quality and outcome of patient care through structured peer review whereby clinicians examine their practices and results against agreed explicit standards and modify their practice where indicated (National Health Service Executive [NHS E], 1996).

Some would suggest that standards should be set before auditing practice (NHS Management Executive; NHS ME, 1991), while others identify the stages of the clinical audit process in the following order:

- select topic and design audit; reason for doing; how going to measure?; cases to be included
- collect data; a systematic review of practice
- analyse findings; identification of problems and possible solutions
- implement improvements in care
- repeat data collection, evaluation and action (Tugwell and Manganelli, 1986; National Centre for Clinical Audit, 1997).

Designing the audit

The aim of this audit was to perform a baseline enquiry to measure the extent of oral problems in cancer patients, current mouth care practices, and staff knowledge. We identified the need to develop two tools: one to collect patient data and one to test staff knowledge.

Patient data collection tool: We had no written standard in the unit on which to base our audit tool and were unable to identify one in the literature. We therefore designed a very simple one, which we piloted on a small sample of patients. Piloting a tool is important for the following reasons: assesses ease of use; allows you to check that you are collecting the correct information; prevents you collecting data then wishing you had asked other questions; assesses reliability of tool if data are collected by several people.

Although this tool gave us some information, it left us with more questions than answers and did not identify the many complexities associated with oral problems in these patients, eg. were patients having certain chemotherapy regimes more likely to have problems? Did the risk of problems increase with each course of chemotherapy? Was there increased risk with any tumour site? Our revised tool was developed and piloted and it appeared to give us the information we required. This tool also incorporated a section for review of medical and nursing documentation.

Staff data collection tool: We were unable to find an existing questionnaire relating specifically to oncology, but found a questionnaire developed by Adams (1996) as part of a study to assess nurses' knowledge of oral care within a medical unit. This questionnaire included most of the topics which the authors had planned to incorporate such as demographic details, training received in oral care, knowledge of oral assessment tools, equipment and solutions for oral care, and drugs that affect the oral cavity. Indeed, it had similar aims and permission was sought to use Adams' (1996) questionnaire, with a positive reply.

A number of changes were made to Adams' (1996) questionnaire in order to take account of the needs of this study. The layout was changed whenever possible to include tick boxes to facilitate easier data analysis and the sequence of questions altered to ensure a logical flow. Full colour pictures of oral problems that were likely to be met in the clinical setting were given to respondents to identify, as was a list of common conditions/words used within oral care.

In order to take account of the needs of this study, a pilot study was carried out to test feasibility, to ensure clarity of instructions and to eliminate any ambiguity of questions. In order not to reduce the eventual sample size, four clinical nurse specialists outside of the unit, but working in cancer care, and who were therefore judged to be typical of the target population, completed a questionnaire. As a result of the pilot study changes were made to some of the questions and instructions on how to complete the questionnaire were added.

Collecting the data

Patient data

A total of 127 patients were interviewed. The sample was opportunistic and consisted of patients present as inpatients on the dates of our visits, and the first twelve patients on each visit to the day case chemotherapy suite. Data were collected on each day of the week, Monday to Friday, to ensure representation across all chemotherapy regimes and tumour sites.

Exclusions

Exclusions were as follows:

Chemotherapy suite day cases: new cases because of their heightened anxiety state and the amount of information they are given on their first visit; patients who refused; patients previously interviewed.

Inpatients: Unconscious; confused; unable to speak English; patients considered by the staff to be too ill/distressed; patient refusal; head and neck patients having radiotherapy because of local damage to the oral mucosa and salivary glands from radiotherapy applied directly to the head and neck area.

Permission for the audit was gained from the member of staff in charge on each shift and an explanation of the purpose of the audit was given. To ensure consistency in data collection one auditor interviewed the patient and the other performed the documentation review. We did not want to extend the length of the patients' visit to the chemotherapy suite and therefore used the natural pauses that occurred during their visit.

Method

Structured interviews were conducted with each patient using the audit tool. This included a physical assessment of the patients' mouths. The interviews were conducted in an examination room in the chemotherapy suite and at the bedside on the ward. A full explanation of the purpose of the audit was given and the patient was given the opportunity to refuse to participate.

Documentation

All nursing and medical documentation was analysed to search for evidence of: assessment of the oral cavity; record of any oral problems; monitoring of these problems; any treatment prescribed and outcomes; any record during this admission or since starting chemotherapy; and drug charts were reviewed to record treatments prescribed.

Staff data

The sample consisted of all registered nurses and healthcare assistants working on the oncology unit at the time. This included staff on the inpatient ward, outpatients' clinic and the chemotherapy suite (staffing levels were low at the time, as a result of sixteen whole-time-equivalent vacancies for staff, five staff long-term sick, and no student nurses). As this was a sensitive area in view of the perceived basic nature of the care being considered, a covering letter was attached assuring respondents that this was not a test but a means of identifying what, if any, educational needs nurses on the oncology unit may have. By using self-completed questionnaires, we were able to offer anonymity and confidentiality.

The aims of the study were discussed with the auditor's manager, senior nurse, and team leaders.

Analysing the data

The sample comprised 127 patients. The breakdown of their characteristics are shown in *Table 5.1*.

Normal oral hygiene routine

The results in *Table 5.2* show how often patients cleaned their teeth. These findings were perhaps the most surprising with only 44% (*n*=56) cleaning their teeth twice a day. This indicated a need to educate patients before commencing their chemotherapy on how to care for their mouth to prevent or reduce the incidence of problems during their treatment.

Table 5.1: Breakdown of patient sample (n=127)		
Characteristic	%	n
Male	45	57
Female	55	70
Inpatients	40	51
Day case chemotherapy	60	76
Own teeth	46	59
Full dentures	31	39
Part dentures	23	29

Table 5.2: Normal hygiene routine (n=127)		
How often do you clean your teeth?	%	n
Once a day	37	47
Twice a day	44	56
Three times a day	8	10
After every meal	4	5
Every two days	3	4
Once a week	2	3
Once a month	1	1
Occasionally	1	1

What do you clean your teeth with?

Table 5.3 shows with what implement patients clean their teeth. The majority of patients used a toothbrush and toothpaste. Of the sixty-eight patients with dentures, 68% (*n*=46) soaked their dentures, 60% (*n*=41) in water alone and 40% (*n*=27) in denture cleaner.

Table 5.3: What do you clean your teeth with?		
Characteristic	**%**	**n**
Toothbrush and toothpaste	79	100
Electric toothbrush and toothpaste	3	4
Toothbrush and water — mostly those with dentures after soaking in steradent	17	22
Toothbrush and bleach	1	1
Also flossed	4	5
Also mouthwash	10	13
Soaking in water	60	76
Soaking in denture cleaner	39	50

Do you have any problems with your mouth?

The results of this are shown in *Figure 5.1*. Each patient was asked about specific problems (*Table 5.4*). The responses ranged from having none of these problems with the mode being three problems. Twenty-five per cent (*n*=32) of patients had three problems, 20% (*n*=25) had two problems, and 6% (*n*=8) stated that they had none of the specified problems. However, on examination, only two of these patients had pink, clean and moist lips, tongue, and mucous membranes, and teeth free from debris and plaque. Of the ninety patients that said they had no problems with their mouth, when they were asked if they had specific problems, 91% (*n*=82) answered yes. There were no differences in the number of symptoms experienced between inpatients and outpatients.

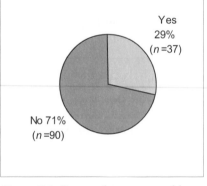

Figure 5.1: Do you have any problems with your mouth?

Have you mentioned these problems to anyone?

The results of this are shown in *Figure 5.2*. When asked why they had not mentioned them to anyone responses included:

> *I expected to have problems.*
> *It was part of the course.*
> *I didn't think anything could be done about it.*

Again this gave us an indication of the need to educate patients to report any problems as early as possible and that there were treatments to relieve symptoms.

Have you ever been given any information on how to look after your mouth? The results of this question are shown in *Figure 5.3*. All patients receiving cytotoxic chemotherapy are advised verbally of the potential effect of this treatment on their mouth and the importance of good oral hygiene. Patients either did not perceive this as information on how to look after their mouth or had forgotten they had been given it.

Table 5.4: Frequency of problems		
Problem	%	n
Altered taste	70	89
Dry lips	68	86
Dry mouth	57	72
Dirty mouth	31	40
Difficulty in swallowing	21	27
Sore mouth	17	21
Problems with teeth	13	16
Sore lips	11	14
Problems with dentures	10	13
Mouth ulcers	9	11
Toothache	7	9
Thrush	3	4

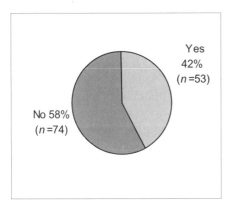

Figure 5.2: Have you mentioned these problems to anyone?

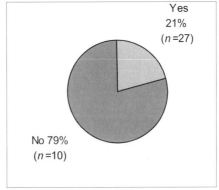

Figure 5.3: Have you ever been given any information on how to look after your mouth?

Patient diagnosis

The sample was representative of a range of solid tumours including breast, lung, prostate, upper gastrointestinal, hepatobiliary, colorectal, and gynaecological. Patients receiving radiotherapy for head and neck cancers were excluded.

From the sample of patients who attended the chemotherapy suite there was no obvious link between oral hygiene problems and site of tumour, the chemotherapy regime used; and the stage of treatment.

Inpatients (40%; n=51) who were identified as having the most oral problems were those admitted with:

- chemotherapy-induced neutropenia (25%; n=13)
- dyspnoea (16%; n=8)
- nausea and vomiting (6%; n=3)

- pain control (16%; $n=8$)
- spinal cord compression (6%; $n=3$).

The first three did not surprise us but the second two led to the assumption that as a result of pain patients did not see oral hygiene as a priority or that these patients were unable to access oral hygiene facilities without assistance.

Documentation

There were inconsistencies in documentation, eg. an oral problem may be mentioned on one day then no further mention made to indicate improvement or deterioration. Of the thirteen patients admitted with chemotherapy-induced neutropenia, less than 50% had their mouths assessed on admission. There were also inconsistencies in prescribing practices in terms of dosage, frequency, and length of treatment.

Comments from patients

Several patients stated that they were just too tired to be bothered to clean their teeth except first thing in the morning. The patients whose only problem was a dry mouth and/or altered taste did not bother to mention these as they seemed trivial and expected it to happen; however, the implications for not treating these are: increased risk of tooth decay as a result of insufficient saliva; increased risk of infection; and decreased appetite resulting in weight loss.

One patient stated that she could not follow her usual routine while in hospital as she was unable to reach the bathroom without assistance and she did not like to ask the nurses for help, as she did not want to bother them. Many patients wished to make it clear that by answering our questions they were not criticising the care they had received and took the opportunity to tell us how well they felt they were being looked after. Some patients offered to help with any further work we would be doing as a result of this study.

Summary of findings

The findings of this study showed that despite oral problems being common they were: underreported by patients; underdiagnosed by doctors and nurses; inadequately treated; and inadequately documented.

Staff knowledge data

A total of forty-two questionnaires to assess staff knowledge were distributed and twenty-six (62%) were returned. The respondents were all female.

What factors do you look for to indicate a healthy mouth?

Out of a possible seven factors (*Table 5.5*), one nurse (4%) could not name any, four (15%) named one, six (23%) identified fresh breath and healthy gums, while no-one mentioned clean, well-fitting dentures.

Name six drugs which adversely affect oral health

Poor knowledge of the effects of drugs on the oral cavity, other than cytotoxics, was displayed (*Table 5.6*). Fifty per cent of nurses (*n*=13) named less than three drugs.

Recognition of common oral problems

Staff were asked to identify photographs of common oral conditions, which included mucositis, xerostomia, mouth ulcer, Candida spp., coated tongue, brown and black hairy tongue, and gingivitis. The nurses showed greater knowledge in this area. A total of twenty-one staff (81%) recognised *Candida* spp., xerostomia, and gingivitis. However, only 50% (*n*=13) were able to identify four of the possible seven conditions presented to them.

Table 5.5: Factors to indicate a healthy mouth

Factor	%	n
Moist mucosa	62	16
Pink mucosa	46	12
Clean teeth	54	14
Pink tongue	50	13
Fresh breath	23	6
Healthy gums	23	6
Well-fitting dentures	0	0

Table 5.6: Drugs that adversely affect the mouth

Drug	%	n
Cytotoxic drugs	85	22
Antibiotics	58	15
Opiates	27	7
Steroids	27	7
Antidepressants	12	3
Diuretics	19	5
Iron	8	2
Antihistamines	8	2
Inhalers	4	1
Hyoscine	4	1
Phenytoin	8	2

None of them were able to identify severe mucositis which, as already mentioned, has major implications for these patients in terms of morbidity and mortality (Berger and Eilers, 1998). Respondents also showed a lack of knowledge of equipment and solutions for oral health care. The literature clearly supports the use of soft toothbrushes (Clarke, 1993; Buglass, 1995; Moore, 1995) and yet only 54% (*n*=14) said this was their tool of choice. The remaining 46% (*n*=12) selected foam applicators and gauze wrapped round a finger as their tools of choice, and sodium bicarbonate as the solution of choice. Some of these, eg. sodium bicarbonate and in some cases foam applicators, have actually been shown to be harmful in oral care (Kite and Pearson, 1995).

A total of eighteen (69%) staff felt that their knowledge of the subject was inadequate but indicated that they would welcome further training. One of the nurses said:

> I thought I had sufficient knowledge until answering the questionnaire.

Only sixteen (62%) of the staff had received any training, either during pre-registration training or subsequently in ENB or NVQ courses. Overall, the knowledge deficits identified in this audit were assessment of the oral cavity, recognition of common problems, knowledge of tools and solutions, and drugs that affect the oral cavity. These findings matched those in Adams' (1996) study except that a significant number of respondents in our survey selected the toothbrush as a tool of choice, 54% (*n*=14) compared with Adams' (1996) finding of 35.3%.

Limitations of the study

The difficulties/constraints in data collection were:

- space in the chemotherapy suite to examine patients' mouths
- concern from patients; they worried that they would miss their chemotherapy slot while they were talking to us
- time; the audit had to be incorporated into our existing workload
- chemotherapy notes were dictated and therefore the record of the consultation was not written in the patients' notes immediately.

Presenting the results

The results of the audit were presented verbally with a written summary for reference. The results were presented to:

- the individual nursing teams within the oncology unit since these were the staff that had participated in the audit
- the oncology audit group meeting which is a multiprofessional group
- other staff within the trust at two nursing study days
- other healthcare groups within leicestershire
- delegates at an international conference.

The results of this study clearly identified service improvements, which were required, including: patient education; staff education; assessment of the oral cavity; and implementing evidence-based care.

Changing practice

Change theory (Bennis *et al*, 1976) identified three strategies:

1. Rational empirical: which assumes people are rational and self-interested and will view change positively as long as they perceive some personal benefits.

2. Power-coercive: which relies on power to direct others requiring only their compliance.
3. Normative-re-educative: which requires participation in change, based on a new understanding of current practices, and a commitment to formulating new approaches. The latter approach fits with the audit cycle as it supports reviewing practices by nursing teams and a problem-solving approach to development (Malby, 1995).

Forces that affect change

According to Malby (1995), the forces that affect change are patients' interests, professions' interests, and organisations' interests. These can be applied to this study.

Patients' interests, being empowered through information: The patients interviewed took a keen interest in the audit findings and were eager to have written information which would allow some element of self-care.

Professions' interests, patient care improves: All staff were helpful, there was no resistance to the audit being carried out. The nursing staff showed a great deal of interest in the audit and our findings. There was evidence of changes in the practices of some staff during the audit study. One junior doctor began to write a separate section in his clerking notes for oral assessment on admission as a result of his interest in our study. The staff that completed the questionnaires were very interested in feedback of the results and in receiving any additional education to increase their knowledge. During our study if we identified oral problems in patients who were not receiving treatment we notified the appropriate nurse/ doctor to ensure action was taken.

Organisations' interests, value for money: The unit pharmacist was interested in the development of guidelines to promote consistency of prescribing. The trust encouraged presentation of the findings to other directorates to share good practice and promote evidence-based practice.

Changes introduced into practice as a result of audit findings

Oral assessment tool (OAT)

The audit clearly showed that patients were not routinely assessed for oral problems. The importance of oral assessment and knowledge of the factors that indicate a healthy mouth are important if adequate oral care is to be provided (McElroy, 1984; Porter, 1994; Holmes, 1996). No OAT was in use at that time, but staff felt an OAT would prompt an assessment and welcomed its introduction.

An OAT was developed by the Research, Audit and Development Group of the hospital following review of existing oral assessment tools produced by Heals (1993), Eilers *et al* (1988) and Jenkins (1989). A tool using the basic framework of Heals (1993), adopted by Freer (2000), was piloted with patients and staff on the oncology unit. Following the pilot, a number of amendments were made. The scoring system was removed as this did not appear to reflect individual patient needs, and additional factors were included to reflect the added risk cancer patients faced from developing oral problems. This oral assessment tool was introduced following a staff training programme.

Guidelines

Guidelines for oral care and treatment were developed in conjunction with the multidisciplinary team. They covered oral assessment, risk factors to oral health, basic oral care for dentate and non-dentate patients, and treatment for common oral problems, including a painful mouth, candidiasis, dry mouth, and halitosis.

Patient information leaflet

During our patient audit some patients, but particularly those on chemotherapy, expressed a desire to be more proactive in their care. A leaflet was developed covering risk factors, mouth care, advice on when to seek help and how to deal with a sore mouth, halitosis, altered taste, and dry mouth. A dry mouth and altered taste were the most common problems experienced by the patients in our study. This leaflet is now given to all chemotherapy and radiotherapy patients before starting treatment.

Patient poster

To encourage patients to carry out regular oral care, posters covering risk factors, oral care procedures and symptoms of oral problems were produced and placed in patient bathrooms and wash areas.

Training programme

An education programme was developed for nursing staff. This has been run as a rolling programme and includes practical as well as theoretical aspects of oral care.

Re-audit

A re-audit was carried out to assess the impact of the changes made one year later. The same method and tool was used to collect data from patients and documentation. The audit of staff knowledge was not repeated, the rationale being that if significant changes had occurred in patient care and treatment this would indicate that staff knowledge and awareness had improved. The findings of the reaudit were as follows:

- the oral assessment tool is used for the majority of inpatients
- The most vulnerable patients (eg. neutropenic) have their oral cavity assessed on admission and thereafter daily and any problems are treated effectively
- all patients are given the mouth care leaflet before commencing chemotherapy or radiotherapy to the head and neck.

Feedback from patients has been very positive and they welcome the information provided, which allows them to participate in their care and to take actions to alleviate oral problems. There is increased reporting by patients of previously ignored problems, thus allowing prompt treatment. Oral problems are now diagnosed and treated adequately. The incidence of oral problems has not decreased significantly but the severity has reduced. There have been improvements in documentation of oral problems, care, and treatment. There has been raised interest and awareness of oral hygiene among the nursing staff.

We have produced a poster that identifies how we used the audit cycle to change practice and demonstrated the impact of these changes. This poster is being displayed at local and national conferences to share our work with others.

Conclusion

Oral problems are prevalent in cancer patients and the effects of cancer treatments on the oral cavity can be a cause of morbidity and mortality in these patients. Assessment of the mouth, early recognition and treatment of common problems, and good oral hygiene are essential to prevent potential life-threatening infections and maintain quality of life. Given the generally poor state of oral health assessment, even in 'high-risk' areas such as oncology, it is clearly time for the nursing profession to adopt and implement oral care routinely.

It has been demonstrated that the audit cycle can be used to measure current practice, to implement change, and to evaluate that change. During this study we increased our own knowledge of oral problems that cancer patients face and the evidence-based care and treatment that is required. We were able to apply our knowledge of the audit process in practice and became more confident in presentation skills to a wide variety of audiences. We recognised the importance of involving the patients as users of the service as well as the multidisciplinary team at each stage of the process. We also learnt not to underestimate the length of time it may take to complete the audit cycle. The use of the oral assessment tool and the patient information leaflet within the oncology unit has become firmly grounded in normal practice with clearly measurable improvements in patient care.

Key points

⌘ Oral problems are prevalent in cancer patients and the effects of cancer treatments on the oral cavity can be a cause of morbidity and mortality in these patients.

⌘ The audit showed that oral problems are common, but are under-reported by patients, underdiagnosed by doctors and nurses, inadequately treated, and inadequately documented. Nursing staff were found to have knowledge deficits.

⌘ Changes to practice as a result of audit findings included the development and implementation of an oral assessment tool and oral care guidelines: patient information leaflets and posters were produced. A staff education programme was introduced.

⌘ A subsequent audit, to complete the audit cycle, revealed significant improvements in the diagnosis and treatment of oral problems and increased reporting of previously ignored problems by patients.

References

Adams R (1996) Qualified nurses lack adequate knowledge related to oral health, resulting in inadequate oral care of patients on medical wards. *J Adv Nurs* **24**: 552–60

Allbright A (1984) Oral care for the cancer chemotherapy patient. *Nurs Times* **80**(21): 40–2

Barnett J (1991) A reassessment of oral healthcare. *Prof Nurse* **6**(12): 703–8

Bennis W, Benne K, Chin R (1976) *The Planning of Change*. 3rd edn. Holt, Reinhart and Winston, London

Berger A, Eilers J (1998) Factors influencing oral cavity status during high dose antineoplastic therapy. *Oncol Nurs Forum* **25**(9): 1623–6

Bowsher J, Boyle S, Griffiths J (1999) Oral care. A clinical effectiveness-based systematic review of oral care. *Nurs Standard* **13**(37): 31

Boyle S (1992) Assessing mouth care. *Nurs Times* **88**(15): 44–6

Buglass E (1995) Oral hygiene. *Br J Nurs* **4**(9): 516–9

Clarke G (1993) Mouth care and the hospitalized patient. *Br J Nurs* **2**(4): 225–7

Coleman S (1995) An overview of the oral complications of adult patients with malignant haematological conditions who have undergone radiotherapy or chemotherapy. *J Adv Nurs* **22**: 1085–91

Crosby C (1989) Method of mouth care. *Nurs Times* **85**(35): 38–41

Department of Health (1989) *Working for Patients*. DoH, London

Department of Health (1999a) *Making a Difference*. DoH, London

Department of Health (1999b) *Continuing Professional Development:Quality in the New NHS*. DoH, London

Department of Health (2001) *Essence of Care*. DoH, London

Driezen S, McCredie KB, Keating MJ (1982) Oral infections associated with chemotherapy. *Postgrad Med* **71**: 133–46

Eilers J, Berger AM, Petersen M (1988) Development, testing and application of the oral assessment guide. *Oncol Nurs Forum* **15**(3): 325–30

Freer SK (2000) Use of an oral assessment tool to improve practice. *Prof Nurse* **15**(10): 635–7

Gibson K, Horsfod J, Nelson W (1997) Oral care: ritualistic practice reconsidered within a framework of action research. *J Cancer Nurs* **4**: 183–90

Hatton-Smith CK (1994) A last bastion of ritualized practice? A review of nurses knowledge of oral healthcare. *Prof Nurse* **9**(5): 304–8

Heals D (1993) A key to wellbeing. *Prof Nurse* **8**(6): 391–8

Henderson V (1960) *The Basic Principles of Nursing Care*. International Council for Nurses, Switzerland

Holmes S (1996) Nursing Management of oral care in older patients. *Nurs Times* **92**(9): 37–9

Howarth H (1977) Mouth Care procedures for the very ill. *Nurs Times* **73**(10): 354–5

Jenkins DA (1989) Oral care in the ICU: an important nursing role. *Nurs Standard* **8**(4): 24–8

Kite K, Pearson L (1995) A rationale for mouthcare: the integration of theory with practice. *Intens Crit Care Nurs* **11**: 71–6

Knox JJ *et al* (2000) Chemotherapy induced oral mucositis, prevention and management. *Drugs Aging* **17**(4): 257–67

Lee L, White B, Ball J *et al* (2001) An audit of oral care practice and staff knowledge in hospital palliative care. *Int J Pall Nurs* **7**(8): 395–400

Lewis IA (1984) Developing a research-based curriculum, an exercise in relation to oral care. *Nurse Ed Today* **3**(6): 143–4

Longhurst RHC (1998) A cross-sectional study of the oral healthcare instruction given to nurses during their basic training. *Br Dent J* **184**(9): 453–7

McElroy (1984) Infection in the patient receiving chemotherapy for cancer: oral considerations. *J Am Dent Assoc* **109**: 454–6

Macmillan Practice Development Unit (1995) *Managing Oral Care Problems throughout the Cancer Illness Trajectory*. Macmillan Cancer Relief and The Royal Marsden NHS Trust, London

Malby B, ed (1995) *Clinical Audit for Nurses and Therapists*. Scuton Press, London

Milligan S, McGill M, Sweeney MP, Malarkey C (2001) Oral care for people with advanced cancer: an evidence-based protocol. *Int J Palliat Nurs* **7**(9): 418–26

Moore J (1995) Assessment of nurse administered oral hygiene. *Nurs Times* **91**(9): 40–1

National Centre for Clinical Audit (1997) *Key Points from Audit Literature Related to Criteria for Clinical Audit*. NCCA, London

NHS E (1996) *Clinical Audit in the NHS. Using Clinical Audit in the NHS: A Position Statement*. NHS E, Leeds

NHS E (1991) *Framework of Audit for Nursing Services*. HMSO, London

Ohrn KEO, Wahlin YB, Sjoden PO (2000) Oral care in cancer nursing. *Eur J Cancer Care* **9**(1): 22–9

Peate I (1993) Nurse administered oral hygiene in the hospitalized patient. *Br J Nurs* **2**(9): 459–62

Pearson LS (1996) A comparison of the ability of foam swabs and toothbrushes to remove dental plaque: implications for nursing practice. *J Adv Nurs* **23**: 62–9

Poland J (1991) Prevention and treatment of oral complications in the cancer patient. *Oncology* **5**(7): 45–62

Porter H (1994) Mouth Care in cancer. *Nurs Times* **90**(14); 27–9

Royal College of Nursing (1996) *Clinical Effectiveness. A Royal College of Nursing Guide*. RCN, London

Rosenberg W, Donald A (1995) Evidence-based Medicine: an approach to clinical problem-solving. *Br Med J* **310**: 1122–6

Trenter Roth P, Creason NS (1986) Nurse administered oral hygiene: is there a scientific basis? *J Adv Nurs* **11**: 323–31

Tugwell P, Mongonelli E (1986) The Clinical Audit Cycle. *Aust Clin Rev* June: 101–5

Walsh H, Ford P (1989) *Nursing Rituals, Research and Related Actions*. Heinemann Nursing, London

White SS (1997) Evidence-based practice and nursing: the new panacea? *Br J Nurs* **6**(37): 175–8

White R J (2000) Nurse assessment of oral health: a review of practice and education. *Br J Nurs* **9**(5): 260–6

6

The importance of oral hygiene in nutritional support

Christine V Jones

Disorders of the mouth can significantly impair the quality of life of the ill patient. For patients requiring nutritional support, especially those who are unable to take food via the oral route, good oral hygiene is of prime importance. This chapter suggests aims and objectives for mouth care plus an assessment tool for recording the oral state of patients on admission. The role of saliva in oral health is explored along with the problems and alleviation of a dry mouth. The current range of oral hygiene products and their use are discussed. A sound scientific knowledge of the oral environment in nurse education is advocated; it is suggested that the dental team could help to provide this.

The importance of a healthy, comfortable mouth in maintaining quality of life is highly relevant to the care of all patients, particularly dysphagic elderly and stroke patients. Feeding/provision of nutrition is not a medical treatment, but a basic human need (Smithard, 1996). Relevant endpoints of nutritional support, functional and clinical outcomes, such as length of stay and improvement in quality of life, should be measured, rather than physiological endpoints such as increase in weight or mid-arm circumference (Allison, 1996). The enjoyment and value of food taken by the enteral route is made possible by careful attention to oral hygiene and oral comfort, which will also improve the quality of life of dysphagic patients.

Attention to oral hygiene is of prime importance to patients who are unable to take food via the oral route, including patients receiving parenteral nutrition (nutrition via the venous route). Bacterial plaque will accumulate in the mouths of these patients as a result of inactivity of the oral structures.

Disorders of the mouth can add significantly to the discomfort, social isolation and distress of ill patients, and severely impair their nutritional intake. Even a minor alteration in the health of the oral cavity can have a significant effect on a person's well-being (Barnett, 1991). Regular mouth care is essential if oral problems are to be prevented (Regnard and Fitton, 1989). Risk factors for reduced oral feeding are listed in *Table 6.1*.

In this decade, scant attention has been paid to the specific relationship between oral care and nutritional intake in the scientific and healthcare literature, although many authors imply that nutritional intake is impaired by lack of attention to oral care (or lack of knowledge of the patient's oral state) (Watson, 1989).

The aims of this chapter are:

- to provide a logical and informed approach to oral care for dependent patients, especially those requiring nutritional support

Table 6.1: Risk factors for reduced oral feeding
Debility
Anorexia
Nausea
Vomiting
Dysphagia
Local tumour
Weakness
Odour
Anticholinergic drugs
Local irradiation
Malignant ulceration
Chemotherapy
Dehydration

- to state aims and outcomes for mouth care
- to offer a simple assessment tool for recording oral findings on admission
- to discuss approaches to routine mouth care
- to recommend suitable products for effective oral hygiene
- to encourage nursing staff to use dental clinicians (dentists, hygienists and dental therapists) to provide regular 'in-house' dental training for nurses, such as that described by Munday and Gelbier (1984).

In an ideal world the dental hygienist has a significant and important role to play in managing patients who need assistance in maintaining oral health. Hygienists can offer clinical knowledge and practical help and thus release nursing staff from this area of care. However, since (in the UK) only 150 of the 3,833 hygienists currently registered with the General Dental Council (The Rolls of Dental Auxiliaries, 2001) are employed in hospital service, this is not feasible at present. Certainly, consideration of such a service should be prioritised, but for the present dental personnel are best used to disseminate knowledge via the in-service training route and when a diagnosis is needed.

Following tradition, and in line with the thinking of Miller and Rubenstein (1987), nurses are the hospital personnel of choice to ensure that all hospitalised patients maintain an acceptable level of routine oral health care and receive dental treatment for acute problems. Nurses should include mouth care as part of daily hygiene for debilitated patients. In addition, nurses can be pivotal in encouraging patients who are capable of self-care to practise effective oral hygiene. In a study of the nurse's role in oral healthcare for hospitalised patients, nurses indicated a high level of interest in improving their ability to offer appropriate oral care services (Miller and Rubenstein, 1987).

It is accepted that oral diseases are the most common diseases in the world. They affect the hard tissues (the teeth), the supporting structures (the periodontium), and the soft tissues (cheeks, tongue, palate, and floor of the mouth). Oral disease affects those who are dentate (having natural teeth) and those who are edentulous (without natural teeth) since patients who have no natural teeth may experience pain and pathology of the oral structures.

Oral cancer is not uncommon in the UK, and about 2500 new cases of malignant tumours of the oral epithelium are reported in England and Wales each year (Levine, 1996). As an argument for regular whole mouth examination, all cases of oral cancer benefit from early diagnosis.

In the last UK Adult Dental Health Survey (Walker and Cooper, 1998),

30% of the dentate adults interviewed said that they only went to the dentist when they had trouble. However, over 500 different bacterial species colonise the mouth, over 400 species live beneath the gum (gingival margin), and 69% of all adults have periodontal disease in one or more sites in their mouth. Only 5% of adults are completely free from clinical signs of inflammation (Moore and Moore, 1994).

These figures suggest that many people will enter hospital with less than healthy mouths. An infinite variety of oral conditions will be present on examination at admission to hospital. Furthermore, diseases such as periodontal disease are recognised risk factors for heart disease and low birthweight in children born to mothers who suffer from one of the many periodontal diseases (Offenbacher *et al*, 1996). It is only by making a baseline assessment of the oral condition and recording this that an informed care plan can be prepared for each individual patient. The aims and objectives of mouth care are listed in *Table 6.2* and a simple oral assessment tool is shown in *Figure 6.1*.

Table 6.2: Aims and objectives of mouth care

Aims of mouth care	Oral comfort and oral health, thereby enhancing the quality of life
Objectives of mouth care	To maintain the oral mucosa and lips, clean, soft, moist and intact
	To keep the natural teeth free from plaque and debris
	To maintain denture hygiene and prevent denture-induced disease
	To prevent infection
	To prevent oral discomfort
	To encourage adequate nutritional intake
	To maintain the mouth in a state of normal function

The verbal history may highlight areas of patient complaint that might otherwise go undetected. It will certainly help in continuity of care, and will assist in maintaining patient dignity in areas such as the patient's desire not to be seen without dentures. Provided that dentures are clean and there is no other contra-indication, they can be retained if that is the patient's habit and desire.

For the intra-oral examination and the handling of dentures, it is essential that the operator wears gloves to prevent cross-infection (particularly the spread of hepatitis B and hepatitis C and human immunodeficiency virus). Noting and attending to dryness and cracking of the lips does a great service to patient comfort. Breaks at the commissures (corners of the lips), which are frequently painful, may indicate a fungal infection (Scully and Cawson, 1982).

Record all findings on case notes. Sit the patient in a good light

Verbal history ⌘ Questions and answers about dental home care:
— does the patient have any oral complaints?
— does the patient wear dentures?
— does the patient wear dentures to sleep in?

Wear gloves for the oral examination!

Extra-oral ⌘ Note condition of lips:
— are they soft, moist (without dribbling) and intact?
— are they dry, cracked, overclosed, crusted at the corners?
⌘ Note any facial asymmetry or lymphadenopathy
⌘ Is the patient pale or cyanosed?
⌘ Does the patient have any visible facial lesions?

Intra-oral — soft tissues ⌘ Ask patient to remove any dentures themselves if possible
⌘ Examine the following using a pen torch, mouth mirror (available in packs of 100 for £17.99 from CTS Dental Supplies) and clean gauze
— cheeks
— tongue (smooth or rough, clean or coated)
— palate (roof of mouth)
— floor of the mouth
— vestibule (inside the lips)
⌘ Are the above pink or naturally pigmented, soft, moist, intact?
⌘ Are they ulcerated, coated or inflamed?
⌘ Are there any white or red patches?
⌘ Does the tongue move freely side to side?
⌘ Is there any pocketing of debris in the cheeks?
⌘ Is there halitosis (bad breath)?

Intra-oral — teeth ⌘ Are there teeth present in upper arch (jaw)?
⌘ Are there teeth present in lower arch?
⌘ Few teeth or many?
⌘ Do they look cared for or neglected, clean or dirty?
⌘ Are they stained?
⌘ Are they generally firm or loose?

Intra-oral — gums ⌘ Are they firm and pink or naturally pigmented?
⌘ Are they inflamed, enlarged or bleeding?

Dentures ⌘ Are these upper, lower or both?
⌘ Are they acrylic or metal or both?
⌘ Are they in good condition, or broken, clean or dirty?
⌘ Is the patient able to control the dentures for speaking and eating?

Figure 6.1: A simple oral assessment tool

Halitosis can be a great barrier to communication between patients and their close relatives and friends. It can generally be dispelled with good, regular oral hygiene and mouth moistening, but it may indicate pathology, which will be revealed on intra-oral examination. Broken, diseased teeth, heavy deposits of plaque and tartar, or bleeding, inflamed gums may be responsible for halitosis, or the cause may be something as simple as putrefying food debris or dirty dentures, for which simple remedies are available (see later). It should be borne in mind that pathology of the respiratory or gastrointestinal tract may be involved. Any bleeding that suggests a blood dyscrasia should be reported.

Neglected teeth can at least be kept clean until a more opportune moment for professional dental care arises. Improvement in oral hygiene may be all that is needed to reduce inflamed gums.

With the information gleaned from the initial examination a personal care plan for the mouth care of the individual patient covering tooth brushing, mouth cleaning and moistening and denture care can be drawn up. How often this should be done is based on need and should be indicated. Where there are problems, repeat examinations can be suggested to check progress.

Use of assessment results

With the aims and outcomes of mouth care in mind, and the information obtained from the initial examination, it should be possible to draw up a care plan for the individual patient under the following headings: lips and soft tissues; moistening; tooth brushing; denture cleaning; and application of medicaments.

In order to understand what deposits other than food need to be removed from the mouth, it is important first of all to look at the formation of plaque and the implications for the patient of allowing it to accumulate in the mouth.

Implications of dental plaque for oral health

Dental plaque is a soft non-calcified microbial deposit which accumulates on the surfaces of the teeth and other firm objects in the mouth, ie. restorations (fillings), dentures, and dental calculus (tartar). It can only be detached by mechanical friction, eg. tooth brushing; it cannot be removed by rinsing or by water sprays. In small amounts it is not visible and its presence can only be revealed by staining with disclosing dyes. In thicker layers it can be seen by the naked eye as a creamy deposit.

The presence of food is not necessary for the formation of plaque, and it continues to form in the mouths of those who are receiving nil by mouth. Dental plaque is the primary cause of the two major dental diseases: dental decay (caries) and periodontal (gum) disease.

Loe *et al* (1965) established that the withdrawal of oral hygiene measures in the mouths of healthy individuals with normal gingivae (gums) resulted in gross accumulations of soft debris and the development of marginal gingivitis in all subjects within a period of ten to twenty-one days. Reinstitution of oral hygiene resulted in the return of healthy gingival conditions.

Plaque is removed by mechanical friction, ie. with toothbrushes, interdental brushes, dental tape and floss. The development of plaque can be inhibited by the use of chlorhexidine gluconate in the form of mouthwash and gel. Methods are discussed in the section on routine mouth care.

Saliva and oral health

An understanding of the role of saliva in dental health will help in the treatment of xerostomia (dryness of the mouth) and its side-effects. Xerostomia is one of the most common side-effects of debilitating illness. In the aetiology of temporary xerostomia, anxiety and depression are well recognised causes of reduced basal flow of saliva (Bates and Adams, 1968). Eating, speaking and denture wearing become difficult and painful, the sensation of taste is diminished, and the natural cleansing mechanism of saliva is lost. In the long term, a reduced salivary flow can result in inflammation and infection, stomatitis, glossitis, cheilitis, mucosal ulcers, dental caries (decay) and candidiasis (thrush) (Sreebny and Valdini, 1987).

In simple terms, the most essential role of saliva is lubrication and protection of the oral mucous membrane. By coating and adsorption onto the mucosa, saliva allows the oral surfaces to move against one another with minimal friction so that speech and taste are possible.

A second mechanical property of saliva is its ability to bind food, enabling it to be formed into a bolus for swallowing (Levine, 1989). Saliva contains many enzymes that are important in the early phase of digestion.

Over 400 commonly prescribed drugs possess the ability to limit salivary flow (Sreebny and Valdini, 1987). In addition, xerostomia can arise from mouth breathing, oxygen therapy, poor appetite, anxiety, general debility, depression, radiotherapy, chemotherapy and diseases of the salivary glands. Some dryness is due to inadequate or total lack of salivary function, and some is simply a 'feeling' of dryness.

Whatever the cause of the xerostomia, attention must be paid to its alleviation if nutritional intake is to be encouraged. This can be achieved by the use of lubricated swabs, mouth rinsing, sipping water, swabbing with crushed ice, and saliva substitutes (see later).

Sores/ulcers due to xerostomia

Sores or ulcers (sometimes called sordes) can occur in dry, inactive mouths when food debris or tablets become attached to the delicate oral mucous membrane. The tissue beneath the debris becomes inflamed and breaks down. Prevention involves regular gentle swabbing to remove the debris before substances become dried on the mucous membrane. The use of an antibacterial gel (chlorhexidine) will aid healing. A surface analgesic such as benzydamine hydrochloride (Difflam) will often reduce the pain.

Halitosis

As stated previously, halitosis can be a barrier between the patient and his/her family. It can also make life difficult for the nursing staff. Masks are a great help with this. However, much of the problem of halitosis can be alleviated by good attention to mouth care.

Mouth care procedures and techniques

Soft tissue cleaning

Lip crusting can be gently removed by sponging with warm water. After drying the lips, a thin film of petroleum jelly should be applied at regular intervals to keep the lips soft and intact. Any breaks in the lips should be investigated and treated. Herpes simplex (cold sores) should be treated with acyclovir cream (Zovirax). Angular cheilitis (thrush at the corners of the mouth) will require treatment with an antifungal ointment, often in conjunction with an antibacterial cream, such as Bactroban, because co-infection by *Candida albicans* and *Staphylococcus aureus* is common.

Intra-oral mucous membrane

Gentle swabbing will remove debris and soften and moisten the oral mucous membrane, helping to keep it intact. This can be done with MOI-STIR swabsticks, which are pH-balanced swabsticks moistened with an aqueous solution containing salivary electrolytes (see later), with pink swabs on sticks moistened with warm water or saline, or with pink swabs on sticks moistened with a thin film of chlorhexidine gel or lightly moistened with chlorhexidine mouthwash (0.2%).

If the tongue is very coated, try gentle swabbing as above, preferably with MOI-STIR swabsticks.

Any candidal infection in the mouth needs treating with an antifungal agent. In the immunocompromised patient it is wise to seek help speedily in the diagnosis and treatment of fungal infections. If in doubt, any unusual appearance in the mouth should be seen by a dentist and/or doctor.

Good personal oral care and an appreciation of the importance of a comfortable, healthy mouth will raise expectations of what can be achieved for those who are dependent on us for providing oral care.

Moisture control in mouth care

Careful use of suction in patients with problems of dysphagia is essential to avoid choking or aspiration of moisture, and limited use of fluids when carrying out mouth care is advised.

If possible, have the patient in an upright position and have a bowl ready for expectoration of saliva, etc.

When possible, work at the side of the patient, cradling the head to give the patient a feeling of security and firmness.

Tooth brushing technique

In the interest of cross-infection control, gloves should always be worn when carrying out mouth care. Remove any partial dentures into a bowl. Begin to work at the front of the mouth in the upper jaw. Use a soft brush, either lightly moistened with water or with a very small amount of toothpaste (or a similar amount of chlorhexidine gel) pressed into the surface of the brush. This prevents paste/gel being dislodged in the mouth and possibly aspirated.

Place the brush sideways against the teeth, overlaying the gum edge with bristles pointing towards the roots of the teeth. Employ a simple side-to-side motion, moving the brush head only a fraction of an inch at a time. This is accurately described as a vibratory movement. Use light pressure, squeezing the gum tissue against the teeth. Move around the upper teeth, replacing the brush section by section against the teeth. Try to use the same action around the inside of the upper jaw.

Do the same on the outer and inner surfaces of the lower jaw, and complete the task by gently scrubbing the occlusal (chewing) surfaces of the upper and lower teeth with a forward and backward motion. This way the mouth is cleaned in sections, and most importantly the plaque is removed from the crevice where gum meets tooth and where it causes inflammation if left.

If possible, get the patient to rinse the mouth with warm water to remove debris, paste, etc. Alternatively, use pink swabs on sticks lightly moistened with saline or warm water to gently sweep away toothpaste and debris.

Denture care

Always wear gloves when handling dentures.

The basic care of any dentures consists of scrubbing with soap and water and soaking in clean water when not worn. It is vital to scrub off debris before dentures are put to soak in any type of proprietary cleaner. Dentures should be removed into a container first and then rinsed to remove any loose debris. Using a brush specifically for the cleaning of that patient's denture, scrub all surfaces over a bowl of tepid water to remove all debris. A denture paste or a little soap can be used and then rinsed away thoroughly. Dentures can be stored when not worn in a marked container filled with clean water.

To reduce the risk of oral candidiasis (thrush), plastic dentures can be soaked two or three times a week in a solution of dilute hypochlorite. Dentural, a proprietary brand of hypochlorite cleaner, makes this easier and instructions for dilution are given on the label. Always rinse dentures thoroughly after soaking in a proprietary cleaner before replacing them in the mouth. Dentures with metal portions and especially chrome cobalt skeleton dentures should only be immersed in dilute hypochlorite for a short time, ie. twenty minutes, because of the danger of corrosion.

Agents and equipment

A vast range of oral hygiene products are available to the consumer. Many are of excellent quality, but the sheer quantity makes selection a problem. However, the choice can be made easier if a few simple rules are followed.

Toothbrushes

Toothbrushes are the tool of choice for removal of dental plaque. Choose small head, flat trim, soft-to-medium texture brushes (nylon or polyester filaments). Good brands have a high degree of finish to each filament.

Wash well and dry after use. Do not store in a toilet bag or container, but allow to dry in the air. Replace every six to twelve weeks.

Dentifrice (toothpaste)

Always choose a fluoridated formulation and a low fluoride formulation for young children. Choose gentle and mild formulations for sick people. Avoid those which bleach the teeth or are very abrasive. Use a small pea-sized amount of paste, pressed down into the brush to avoid accidental ingestion of the paste.

Small children should be supervised when brushing to prevent swallowing of the paste, which can lead to ingestion of too much fluoride and result in mottling or fluorosis of the permanent dentition.

Bicarbonate of soda was traditionally used to cleanse mouths because of its ability to break down mucin in the mouth. For the same reason, baking soda toothpaste makes the mouth feel squeaky clean and may be preferred by some patients. However, caution is urged with the use of sodium bicarbonate with critically ill patients as it may cause electrolyte imbalance. Generally speaking, toothpaste has a drying effect in already dry mouths and should be used sparingly.

Interdental cleansers

Interdental brushes, floss and dental tape should be purchased at the direction of the dentist or hygienist who has assessed the area for cleaning.

Mouthwashes

Most antiseptic mouthwashes, apart from those containing chlorhexidine gluconate, are of limited value as they have only a transient effect. Those containing chlorhexidine gluconate such as Corsodyl, Chlorhex and Eludril are valuable in reducing the bacterial count by up to 80% (Schiott *et al*, 1970). They are adsorbed onto the epithelium and tooth surface and released over seven hours or so if used as a rinse for one minute. This form of chemical plaque control is of particular value in nursing the sick and immunocompromised patient and the frail elderly. Side-effects include staining of the teeth. Chlorhexidine gluconate mouthwash can also be used on swabs or in gel form if the patient is unable to control fluids in the mouth.

In general, mouthwashes are alcohol-based and for this reason can cause discomfort if the oral mucosa is broken. However, chlorhexidine gluconate mouthwashes are extremely effective for their antibacterial and fungicidal properties and beneficial in the treatment and prevention of oral conditions. Corsodyl may be diluted 50/50 with water if patients complain of soreness on use of the full-strength mouthwash; the diluted preparation will still retain a proportion of the efficacy of the full-strength preparation.

Fluoride mouthwashes are useful in the treatment of tooth sensitivity, in the remineralisation of the early carious lesion, and in reducing the risk of dental decay (Kidd and Joyston-Bechal, 1987). They are not advised for children under the age of six years and must be used under supervision with older children. They are unsuitable for patients with dysphagia. They are used daily at 0.05% concentration and weekly at 0.2% concentration.

Surface analgesics

Benzydamine hydrochloride (Difflam) is a locally acting analgesic and anti-inflammatory agent. It can be used for the treatment of soreness in the mouth and is suggested for use before eating to make the process more comfortable.

Lignocaine gel (lignocaine hydrochloride BP 2% m/V with chlorhexidine gluconate solution BP 0.25%V/V) can be used as a surface anaesthetic. Caveat — this is contraindicated where there are cardiac disorders.

Mouth swabs

MOI-STIR pH-balanced swabsticks are excellent for gentle mouth cleaning of the intra-oral surfaces and the alleviation of dry mouth; they act by replenishing moisture content and replacing salivary electrolytes. The salivary supplement in MOI-STIR swabsticks consists of an aqueous solution of electrolytes with sorbitol and sodium carboxymethylcellulose, making them more acceptable than animal-based salivary substitutes. Their neutral pH means that they are far superior to the traditionally used glycerin and lemon swabs which, because of their acidic nature, can cause demineralisation of the tooth surface. They are presented in a sealed pack of three. Their superiority in terms of patient acceptance has been demonstrated by Poland (1987) in a prospective, randomised, double-blind crossover study with oncology patients.

Pink swabsticks can feel like sandpaper to the delicate oral tissues, but if coated with Corsodyl gel they become more acceptable and will cleanse and confer an antibacterial layer on the mucosa when used for intra-oral swabbing.

Saliva substitutes

Several saliva substitutes are available for the relief of dry mouth:

* Saliva Orthana is a saliva substitute based on natural mucin of animal origin. It is superior for dentate patients as it contains fluoride but is unsuitable for patients whose religion forbids the use of certain animal products.
* Saliveze is an artificial saliva mouth spray of neutral pH containing salivary electrolytes in an aqueous solution with carboxymethylcellulose.
* Glandosane is another artificial saliva.
* Luborant is a saliva substitute containing fluoride.

Of these four saliva substitutes only Luborant is licensed for use in any condition giving rise to a dry mouth (the others having ABCS approval for dry mouth associated with radiotherapy or sicca syndrome) (*British National Formulary*, 1996).

Conclusion

Disorders of the mouth may significantly impair nutrition via the enteral route; therefore, every effort should be made to maintain mouths in a state of comfort and health. Much is to be gained by careful attention to oral cleanliness and comfort.

Universal mouth care policies and packs do not provide for the needs of individual patients because of their inflexibility. Care plans should be devised for each individual patient based on the findings of the baseline examination, and be regularly updated. Mouth care products should be obtained as necessity indicates.

If effective mouth care based on sound scientific principles is to be provided, there needs to be recognition of the need for in-service training of nursing staff by dental staff.

Key points

⌘ Good oral hygiene is essential for quality of life, and is of prime importance in the care of those requiring nutritional support.

⌘ A baseline assessment of the mouth will provide essential information for planning personalised mouth care.

⌘ An understanding of the oral environment based on sound scientific knowledge will improve the standard of care given.

⌘ For nurse education in mouth care, the dental team should be used where possible.

References

Allison S (1996) Relevant endpoints of nutritional support. *Clin Nutr Update* **6**(3): 4

Barnett J (1991) A reassessment of oral health care. *Prof Nurse* **6**(12): 703–8

Bates JF, Adams D (1968) The influence of mental states on the flow of saliva. *Arch Oral Biol* **13**: 593–6

British National Formularly (1996) British Medical Association and Royal Pharmaceutical Society of Great Britain, London

Kidd EAM, Joyston-Bechal S (1987) *Essentials of Dental Caries: The Disease and its Management*. Wright, Bristol: 94

Levine RS (1989) Saliva. *Dental Update* **16**(3): 102

Levine R (1996) *The Scientific Basis of Dental Health Education*. 4th edn. Health Education Authority, London: 3, 26

Loe H, Theilade E, Jensen SB (1965) Experimental gingivitis in man. *J Periodontol* **36**: 177–87

Miller R, Rubenstein L (1987) Oral health care for hospitalized patients: the nurse's role. *J Nurs Educ* **26**(9): 362–6

Moore WEC, Moore LVH (1994) The bacteria of periodontal disease. *Periodontology 2000* **5**: 66–77

Munday P, Gelbier S (1984) Provision of dental health education in nurse training. *Nurse Educ Today* **3**(6): 124–5

Offenbacher S, Katz V, Festik G *et al* (1996) Periodontal infection as a possible risk factor for pre-term low birth weight. *J Periodontol* **67**(10): 1103–13

Poland JM (1987) Comparing Moi-Stir to lemon-glycerine swabs. *Am J Nurs* **87**(4): 422–4

Regnard C, Fitton S (1989) Mouth care: a flow diagram. *Palliat Med* **3**: 67–9

Schiott CR, Loe H, Jensen SB, Kilian M, Davies RM, Glavind K (1970) The effect of chlorhexidine mouthrinses on the human oral flora. *J Periodontol Res* **5**: 84–9

Scully C, Cawson SA (1982) Immunodeficiency and immuniologically mediated disease. In: Scully C, Cawson SA, eds. *Medical Problems in Dentistry*. Wright, Bristol: 390–1

Smithard D (1996) The importance of managing dysphagia. *Clin Nutr Update* **6**(3): 2

Sreebny LM, Valdini A (1987) Xerostomia — a neglected symptom. *Arch Intern Med* **147**: 1333–7

The Rolls of Dental Auxiliaries (1995) Published by the General Dental Council, December

Walker A, Cooper I (1998) *Adult Dental Health Survey of the United Kingdom*. HMSO, London

Watson R (1989) Care of the mouth. *Nursing* **3**(44): 20–4

7

Dysphagia: the management and detection of a disabling problem

Lin Perry

Dysphagia represents a varying group of swallowing difficulties commonly encountered in patients in both acute and community settings. It accompanies a variety of disease states, can be neuromuscular or mechanical/obstructive in origin and encompasses varied prognoses and outcomes. Its consequences include dehydration, malnutrition, bronchospasm, airways obstruction, aspiration pneumonia and chronic chest infection, social isolation, depression and detrimental psychosocial effects. Current 'best evidence' in screening, assessment and management is of variable quality but demonstrates that nurses have an important role to play in interventions entailing multiprofessional collaboration within individually tailored programmes. Clear benefits for patients have been indicated. There are gaps in the knowledge base, especially in relation to psychosocial effects and treatment strategies and the nursing contribution in this area.

Food and eating are central to all our lives, not only as a life-support mechanism but also food consumption structures culture, characterises social relationships and contributes to personal identity (Mennell *et al*, 1992). Consequently, anything which affects the ability to eat potentially exerts profound influences in addition to the effect upon nutritional intake.

The consequences of dysphagia have been described as 'refusing to eat in public, fear of swallowing, depression and loss of the joy of eating' (Rosenbek, 1995). At the extreme, it may preclude eating. As well as detrimental psychosocial effects, it may result in dehydration and malnutrition, aspiration pneumonia, bronchospasm and asphyxia.

This potentially distressing situation is not rare. In a random sample of people aged fifty to seventy-nine years from a city census, 35% reported symptoms of dysphagia (Lindgren and Janzon, 1991). Kayser-Jones and Pengilly (1999) found clinical evidence of dysphagia in 55% of nursing home residents described as poor eaters.

Nurses' responsibility to ensure that patients' nutritional needs are met has been emphasised (UKCC, 1997). Consequently, dysphagia has implications for nursing care in many settings. However, as dysphagia derives from a range of causes, it encompasses a variety of signs and symptoms.

The functional swallowing mechanism

Swallowing is commonly described as comprising four phases:

- oral preparatory
- oral
- pharyngeal
- oesophageal (Zorowitz and Robinson, 1999).

Oral preparatory

The first stage entails reception of food or fluid within the mouth and its preparation for swallowing. If chewing is required, control of the bolus must be maintained as it is compressed against the hard palate, then moved laterally and rotated by movements of the tongue and mandible as it is mixed with saliva. Neuromotor control of the lower jaw, tongue, cheek muscles and lips (in combination with tongue tip to prevent leakage from the mouth) are required. Before initiation of swallowing proper, a cohesive bolus is formed.

Oral

During the oral phase the bolus is moved from the oral cavity to the pharynx. The soft palate lifts and combines with constriction of its side walls to block the nasopharynx. The pharynx opens and the posterior tongue is depressed; this forms a chute along which the bolus moves in response to wavelike muscular movement from the anterior tongue along the hard palate.

Pharyngeal

As food enters the oropharynx, the third (pharyngeal) stage of swallowing is initiated entailing a rapid and ordered sequence of actions. While the two previous phases are amenable to voluntary control, much of the third stage is initiated automatically. Mandibular muscles stabilise the base of the tongue as it moves the bolus backwards. The larynx and hyoid bone elevate and pharyngeal constrictor muscles contract as part of a peristaltic wave; pressure in the upper pharynx rises while in the lower segment it falls.

Airway protection is supplied by sequential closure of vocal cords, false vocal cords, lower laryngeal vestibule and final horizontal folding of the epiglottis over the laryngeal inlet; breath-holding is automatic at this point. The cricopharyngeal muscle relaxes as the bolus moves downwards with the peristaltic wave of contraction. Thereafter, the soft palate moves back to its original position; larynx and nasopharynx reopen and respiration restarts (Zorowitz and Robinson, 1999).

Oesophageal

The final oesophageal phase entails the transport of the bolus through the oesophagus to the stomach. This needs ordered and coordinated muscular contractions to move the bolus through the upper striated and lower smooth muscle of the oesophagus and the muscular ring of the oesophageal outlet (Groher, 1997; Logemann, 1998).

With ageing, changes occur in the sensory and motor components of swallowing (Robbins *et al*, 1992; Aviv *et al*, 1994). However, as many diseases associated with dysphagia are more common in older age-groups, disease-related and age-associated effects may occur simultaneously (Feinberg, 1996). It is suggested that age-effects represent a loss of functional reserve, rendering older people more vulnerable to disease-effects (Feinberg, 1996; Hudson *et al*, 2000).

The dysfunctional swallowing mechanism

A wide-range of disease conditions of neurogenic or mechanical/obstructive origin may result in dysphagia (*Table 7.1*). Symptoms may also be treatment-related. Aside from mechanical and obstructive sequels of cancer surgery and radiotherapy, drug-effects and side-effects may also result in swallowing problems:

- extrapyramidal motor symptoms
- anticholinergic-derived reduction in salivation
- corticosteroid-related myopathy
- sedation-effects.

Dysphagia may also be psychogenic in origin. Groher (1997) describes this as a 'diagnosis of exclusion' — only made when all other possibilities have been ruled out.

In neurogenic dysphagia, failure of central or peripheral sensory and/or motor control produces a predominance of oropharyngeal symptoms at presentation. These include slowed or lost coordination or control of the activities required to prepare food and fluid for swallowing and/or disturbance of the swallowing process (*Table 7.2*).

Poor bolus control may be indicated by coughing before swallowing or may produce acute airways obstruction. Poor laryngeal control may be revealed by coughing during swallowing; incomplete clearance of food or fluids from the pharynx results in residues pooling in the throat which may be indicated by throat clearing, a wet-sounding voice or coughing after swallowing although this may not be immediate. Laryngeal penetration (material reaching the level of the vocal cords) and bronchial aspiration (food or fluids beyond the level of the cords) may occur.

Oesophageal symptoms include a sense of food sticking in the throat and regurgitation. However, dysphagia may also be clinically 'silent', resulting in chronic chest infection or acute aspiration pneumonia (Zorowitz and Robinson, 1999).

Table 7.1: Some causes of dysphagia

Neuromuscular problems	Stroke, hemispheric and brainstem Cerebrovascular/Alzheimer's disease Motor neurone disease Multiple sclerosis Traumatic brain injury Cerebral tumours Parkinson's disease Cerebral palsy Central nervous system infections, eg. meningitis Guillain-Barré syndrome and other polyneuropathies Achalasia Myopathies: metabolic, endocrine, muscular dystrophies
Mechanical/ obstructive causes	Head, neck and mediastinal tumours Iatrogenic: fibrosis/mucositis/radionecrosis; following radiotherapy; surgical resection Retropharyngeal infections; tonsillitis Pharyngoesophageal diverticula Intubation: endotracheal; tracheostomy Trauma Dental caries Xerostomia Prominent anterior cervical osteophytes Chronic gastroesophageal reflux

Source: Groher (1997); Zorowitz and Robinson (1999)

Table 7.2: Possible indicators of dysphagia

Drooling and loss of lip seal
Impaired chewing, poor control of food in the mouth
Pocketing of food between cheek and gum, mouth odour
Difficulty initiating swallowing
Delayed or slow swallowing
Nasal regurgitation
Coughing or choking
Residues pooling in the throat resulting in coughing, throat clearing or wet-sounding voice
Food sticking in the throat
Regurgitation, heartburn or chest pain
Chronic chest infection or acute aspiration pneumonia
Weight loss

Source: Zorowitz and Robinson (1999)

The most common cause of neurogenic dysphagia is stroke (Kuhlemeier, 1994). Stroke-related symptoms have been described by Axelsson *et al* (1984), Carr and Hawthorn (1988a, b), and McLaren (1997). However symptoms overlap between diseases; similar effects may be produced by various means. Many of the symptoms of neurogenic dysphagia are also seen where the cause is mechanical or obstructive.

In this situation, where central and some or most local control mechanisms remain intact, function may be impeded or prevented by absence or obstruction of the functional component. For example, inability to manage secretions, manifesting as drooling, may result from loss of neuromuscular control or obstruction by acute pharyngeal infection; tumour or abscess may block food passage through the pharynx, as may the inability to relax the cricopharyngeus following stroke (Logemann, 1998).

Presentation, however, may differ. Dysphagia may be an anticipated effect of known chronic disease (eg. motor neurone disease or metastatic malignancy) or it may occur as a presenting symptom. In both cases full clinical assessment is the first stage. Stroke, however, is slightly different.

Dysphagia screening

Dysphagia is a common accompaniment of stroke, with up to 67% of stroke patients reported affected when screened during the first seventy-two hours (Hinds and Wiles, 1998). Dysphagia is commonly, but not exclusively, associated with increased stroke severity (Perry and McLaren, 2000a); it may occur without other visible stroke symptoms (Celifarco *et al*, 1990). Consequently, it is recommended that all stroke patients are screened for clinical evidence of dysphagia as soon as possible after presentation using a simple validated bedside testing protocol (Intercollegiate Working Party for Stroke for the Royal College of Physicians of London, 2000).

The validity and reliability of published screening tools has been explored (Perry and Love, 2001). The gag reflex is specifically excluded because of its unreliability as a single indicator and its insensitivity with stroke patients (Bleach, 1993; Leder, 1996; Daniels *et al*, 1997). When implemented as part of a nutrition management package, nurse-initiated screening for dysphagia in patients with acute stroke has demonstrated beneficial outcomes (Odderson *et al*, 1995; Perry and McLaren, 2000b).

Where neurogenic dysphagia might be anticipated, eg. in known neurological disease, the essence of effective management is vigilance for symptoms (Groher, 1997). Investigation of screening procedures in neurological disorders other than stroke is warranted.

Clinical assessment of dysphagia

The procedure for clinical assessment of swallowing has been described (Logemann, 1998). It has been incorporated in outline within speech and language therapists' (SLTs') consensus clinical guidelines (Royal College of Speech and Language Therapists, 1998). There is little work evaluating the performance of assessment schedules or how assessment affects outcomes, although Smithard *et al* (1997, 1998) compared SLT assessments with incidence of aspiration seen on videofluoroscopic swallowing studies (VSS) in stroke patients.

Compared to aspiration seen on VSS, the SLT assessments demonstrated sensitivity 47% and specificity 86%. Assessments by two doctors achieved sensitivity 68% or 70%, specificity 67% or 60%. The agreement of the two SLTs' assessments achieved a kappa coefficient of 0.79 (designated 'good agreement'; Landis and Koch, 1977) and that of two doctors produced 0.5 ('moderate agreement'; Smithard *et al*, 1997), while agreement between SLT and doctor only reached a kappa rating of 0.48 ('moderate agreement'). Differences in the aims and timing of the different professional assessments and the variability of swallow function in acute stroke must be borne in mind.

Videofluoroscopic swallowing studies (VSS)

The VSS (also described as a modified barium swallow) entails video filming fluoroscopic images of patients chewing and swallowing a variety of foods impregnated with barium. It has long been regarded as the 'gold standard' assessment, but it has limitations (*Table 7.3*).

Table 7.3: Limitations of videofluoroscopy (VSS)

VSS requires patients to be transported to a radiology department and specifically positioned; even with specially adapted chairs this is not possible for all patients
The procedure is labour-intensive, requiring a minimum of two practitioners
The procedure entails radiation exposure
The procedure entails chewing a range of barium impregnated foods; there is limited standardisation between hospitals of food, fluid and barium volumes, consistencies and textures to be used
In assessing video films of swallowing there is variety in the anatomical landmark movements and duration of movements which are used as criteria of normal swallowing
VSS may not identify problems as they present in the clinical setting, where patients may sit poorly positioned and eat unassisted textures and quantities of foods not used at VSS

Source: Perry and Love, 2001

It is at best a 'snap-shot' view undertaken in unnatural surroundings; this is highlighted by description of a group experiencing 'apraxia of swallowing' with VSS but able to eat in everyday life (Robbins *et al*, 1993).

While no clinical assessment matches the sensitivity or specificity of VSS for abnormal swallowing characteristics or aspiration, the clinical significance of discrepancies is not clear; or to what extent significant problems are overlooked clinically or variant function seen with VSS labelled as problems.

VSS reports consist of judgements depicting the relative normality of filmed swallows and whether or not penetration/aspiration was observed. Reliability of VSS reports has been variously assessed. Daniels *et al* (1997) used a dysphagia severity score and found overall 66% agreement between two independent scorers, and 92% agreement in distinguishing normal/minor abnormality from moderate/ severe dysphagia. Subsequent evaluations demonstrated progressive improvement: 95% interrater agreement (with intrarater scores achieving 80% or 98%), rising to 98% interrater agreement. This possibly illustrates a 'learning curve' within this clinical team (Daniels *et al*, 1997, 1998, 1999).

In a more detailed study using nine raters and swallowing studies of twenty patients (all viewed twice), a range of components of swallowing, penetration and aspiration was investigated (Kuhlemeier *et al*, 1998). A wide range of results was achieved across the consistencies studied, with no consistent patterns revealed between inter- and intrarater comparisons. However, absence of aspiration was a highly reliable observation, as was the presence of aspiration on thin but not thick liquids.

Others have reported different findings. Daniels *et al* (1997, 1998) found presence/absence of both overt and silent aspiration on any consistency achieved 100% agreement. Smithard *et al* (1998) reported 76% agreement, a kappa coefficient of only 0.48. Reportage both within and between groups is clearly variable.

New interventions that will produce relevant and reliable information without the disadvantages seen in *Table 7.3* are actively sought. The combination of bedside clinical assessment with pulse oximetry to detect desaturation on swallowing has demonstrated good sensitivity and specificity for aspiration and penetration seen on VSS and subsequent development of pneumonia during hospital stay (Smith *et al*, 2000; Lim *et al*, 2001). Other options, for which there are presently no rigorous evaluation studies, include cervical auscultation (Stroud, 1997), videoendoscopy (Bastian, 1991), manometry (Perie *et al*, 1998) or the Repetitive Oral Suction Swallow Test (Nilsson *et al*, 1998). Recent evaluation of fibreoptic endoscopic evaluation of swallowing (FEES) and FEES with sensory testing (FEEST) appears promising (Aviv, 2000; Aviv *et al*, 2000).

Dysphagia management

Surgical interventions, resection and stent implantation, may be entailed in management of malignant disease, but these approaches will not be addressed in this chapter. In most cases dysphagia is managed by direct and/or indirect swallowing therapies, dietary manipulation or artificial nutrition support (*Table 7.4*). Nurses have a key role to play in each category.

VSS has value in dysphagia management both in identification of specific dysfunctions and evaluation of the effects of therapeutic manoeuvres (Sorin *et al*, 1988; Martin-Harris *et al*, 2000). This is highlighted by the identification by Daniels *et al* (1997) of thirteen patients with silent aspiration during VSS with liquid barium, nine of whom had coughed with water. This may be explained as a consequence of the variability of swallow function in acute stroke and/or it may demonstrate that by thickening the fluid (barium compared with water), overt dysphagia had been converted to silent aspiration, highlighting potential risks incurred with empirical prescription of 'safe' consistencies.

Table 7.4: Management of dysphagia	
Direct stategies	Stimulation Exercises Medication
Indirect (compensatory) strategies	Supraglottic swallowing Mendelson's manoeuvre Double swallow Head and neck positioning: chin-down posture effect; lateral head rotation Palatal prosthetic devices Size and timing of mouthfuls presented Modification of textures/consistencies of food/fluids
Artificial nutrition	Tube feeding, eg. nasogastric, percutaneous endoscopic gastrostomy, parenteral nutrition

Direct therapies

The aim of direct therapies is restoration of voluntary motor activity. A number of approaches have been described (*Table 7.4*). Stimulation of motor activity and speed of response have been sought by tapping or stretching the area, or applying thermal (cold), electrical and chemical (sour tastes) stimuli (Lazzara *et al*, 1986; Logemann *et al*, 1995; Park *et al*, 1997; Freed *et al*, 2001). Evaluation of these approaches has been limited and benefits have not been demonstrated conclusively, especially in relation to sustainability.

Exercises tailored to specific impairments of tongue, lips, jaw, palate and larynx are frequently recommended (Logemann, 1998). Again, there has been little evaluation of their contribution to swallowing rehabilitation. However, where they have been prescribed by dysphagia-trained therapists, appropriately trained nurses may use them, eg. thermal and chemical stimulation, during meals and all nurses have a role in encouraging and reinforcing exercise regimes. A single study has explored the potential of drug therapy (nifedipine), demonstrating possible benefit, but further work is required to evaluate its contribution to clinical practice (Perez *et al*, 1998).

Indirect (compensatory) strategies

In this case, the aim is to provide compensation via individually tailored interventions. These range from the broad based (eg. ensuring adequate analgesia before eating with painful mucositis, and sipping carbonated liquid between mouthfuls in obstructive dysphagia) to those targeted at specific dysfunction.

In the latter category, supraglottic swallowing was originally developed for patients with partial laryngectomy. Breath is held before swallowing, aiming to adduct the vocal cords and protect the airway. The patient swallows twice and immediately after swallowing must cough to expel anything which has penetrated the laryngeal vestibule (Groher, 1997). However, videonaso-endoscopy has shown that breath-holding does not always result in closed vocal cords. Additionally, concerns have been raised about unwanted cardiovascular effects of this manoeuvre in stroke patients (Chaudhuri *et al*, 2000).

Mendelson's manoeuvre entails deliberate prolonging of laryngeal elevation during mid-swallow, useful if the swallow is weak and the larynx poorly elevating. The aim is to increase the proportion of the bolus going into the oesophagus and to decrease pharyngeal residues (Kahrilas *et al*, 1991). A double swallow may be recommended to improve clearance of food pooled in the pharynx.

Different positions of the head and neck may be suggested to address different problems (Logemann, 1998). The chin-down position shifts the epiglottis backwards with significant narrowing of the laryngeal entrance and increased airway protection. This may be valuable if the pharyngeal phase is delayed, but it does not eliminate aspiration in all patients (Shanahan *et al*, 1993). Lateral head rotation may be useful for those with unilateral paralysis. Rotation opens the upper oesophageal sphincter and moves the bolus away from the paralysed side. This results in easier bolus transit and excludes the flaccid oesophageal sidewall which otherwise dissipates the pressure build-up necessary to move the bolus. As a result, more of the bolus moves and transit is faster, resulting in a greater proportion swallowed with less remaining in the pharynx (Logemann *et al*, 1989). Palatal prostheses have been used to reshape the oral cavity in such a way as to address individual problems in bolus manipulation and trigger swallowing (Logemann, 1998).

Possibly, the most common compensatory strategy entails modification of textures and/or consistencies of food and fluids in accordance with difficulties encountered. With neurogenic dysphagia where bolus control may be defective, the greatest challenge may be posed by thin fluids, foods of multiple textures or food which fragments; thickened fluids and foods with uniform pastelike textures may be safer. In obstructive dysphagia thin fluids may pose no problem while thick or fibrous foods may be unmanageable.

A number of grading schemes have been devised for food and fluid textures and consistencies. Penman and Thomson (1998) reviewed eleven texts detailing between one and five grades for both food and fluids. A lack of standardisation poses problems and is also an issue in clinical practice. The aim is to provide a diet which is appropriate to the type and severity of dysphagia in minimising risks of aspiration or obstruction, meets nutritional requirements and is acceptable to the patient. Ensuring varied, appetising, ethnically acceptable, and nutritious adequate texture-modified diets can pose challenges, and nurses have a role in liaising with hospital caterers, nursing homes, carers and meals-on-wheels providers and in monitoring and providing feedback (Groher, 1997; Stratton *et al*, 1998).

Additionally, many patients will require assistance to eat, and feeding a dysphagic patient is a skilled procedure. The meal environment requires attention.

The atmosphere should be calm and quiet to reduce distraction, and assistance should be provided in an unhurried manner by someone sitting with them. Patients need to be positioned properly (seated upright, adequately supported) with the meal placed where they can see and smell it. Food of the appropriate temperature and texture should be presented in manageable-sized pieces; many cope better with teaspoon-sized morsels presented slowly. The way that food and fluid is presented may be as important as its texture and consistency; Kuhlemeier *et al* (2001) showed that aspiration risk could worsen when some patients drank from cups rather than by spoon.

Prescribed swallowing manoeuvres should be reinforced, eg. double swallow, chin tuck and so on, and the feeder should watch for development of fatigue and deteriorating swallowing function. Cheek pouches should be checked for pocketing (Hargrove, 1980; Hotaling, 1990; Layne, 1990; Sidenvall and Ek, 1993; Van Ort and Phillips, 1995; Wykes, 1997).

Assessment and monitoring of patients' nutritional needs includes ability to eat and is an important responsibility of qualified nurses; activities may be appropriately delegated (UKCC, 1997). The nursing contribution has been shown to be crucial, with staffing directly affecting patients' nutritional intake (Kayser-Jones and Schell, 1997). Recent initiatives have included educational preparation for an expanded nursing role, including assessment and management of patients with minor degrees of dysphagia (Davies *et al*, 2001).

Prediction of therapeutic efficacy of strategies for the individual may be difficult. There is currently no evidence that swallow therapies reduce end-of-therapy dysphagia, although non-compliance with therapeutic prescription has been associated with increased adverse outcomes such as hospitalisation and chest infection (Bath *et al*, 2000; Low *et al*, 2001).

Artificial nutrition support

If adequate dietary intake cannot be achieved orally, enteral feeding may be initiated via finebore nasogastric or nasoenteral tube (usually short-term only), gastrostomy or jejunostomy. If the gastrointestinal tract is non-functional, parenteral nutrition via the central or peripheral route are alternatives. It may also be employed for gut inaccessibility, which may occur when dysphagia precludes eating and nasoenteral tubes are unable to be placed or tolerated (British Society of Gastroenterology, 1996). In this situation, siting of percutaneous endoscopic gastrostomy (PEG) tubes may be preferred, but where there is delay and concern for the patient's nutritional status, parenteral nutrition via the peripheral route may be appropriate (Payne-James and Khawaja, 1993).

Artificial feeding is not without risks. The decision to initiate it should be based on (ideally) the informed views of the patient, clinical information about the patient's prognosis and the progress and likely duration of dysphagia, assessment of risks versus benefits and other factors. Its implementation may be initiated on a limited-time basis to allow evaluation of response to treatment. However, it is important to intervene early to prevent nutritional deterioration (Lennard-Jones, 1998; British Medical Association [BMA], 1999).

Fine-bore nasogastric tubes have been shown to provide a useful short-term means through which to deliver artificial nutritional support. They may be inserted by trained nursing staff, and placement can be checked by gastric aspirate in up to 95% of cases (Neumann *et al*, 1995; Rollins, 1997). However, a proportion of patients (21%; Norton *et al*, 1996) will be unable to tolerate them and inadvertent removal and/or tube blockage may result in significant loss of prescribed feed volume (Park *et al*, 1992).

Feeding via PEG achieves superior feed delivery, with patient and staff preference (Park *et al*, 1992; Norton *et al*, 1996). However, the procedure carries associated morbidity and mortality. Also, it is not clear at what point a PEG should be inserted and follow-up, including recognition of recovery of swallowing, is frequently inadequate (Davies *et al*, 1998; Rehman and Knox, 2000). Neither nasogastric nor PEG feeding abolish the aspiration risk, indeed, they may increase it (Finucane and Bynum, 1996).

Psychosocial considerations

Evidence in relation to 'best practice' is of varied standard. In many areas, too few good quality studies have been undertaken to provide strong evidence to guide management (Bath *et al*, 2000). However, the area most deficient in evidence is that outlined at the beginning; food and eating are central to human society and the impact of dysphagia is anecdotally acknowledged (Rosenbek, 1995; Groher, 1997).

Rickman (1998) has indicated that initiation of PEG feeding may have wide-ranging effects but little work has been undertaken to explore psychosocial consequences across the spectrum of dysphagia or the sequelae of other management strategies. This represents important omissions in an area in which nursing support is either not being evaluated or where nursing intervention might achieve benefit.

Conclusion

The term dysphagia encompasses a broad symptom-category, incorporating differing causes, courses and possible outcomes. It is commonly encountered in both acute and community settings.

On the basis of the current 'best available evidence', the range of options has been outlined, and important gaps in knowledge highlighted. It is clear that dysphagia is an important problem for a substantial group of patients; it is equally important for their nurses.

Key points

⌘ Dysphagia is commonly encountered in both acute and community settings.

⌘ Consequences include starvation and dehydration, aspiration and chest infection, psychological and social disablement.

⌘ Neuromuscular and/or mechanical/obstructive causes produce an array of symptoms which may be clinically 'silent'.

⌘ Early detection and full assessment are important first steps, with a range of treatment options available to meet individual requirements.

⌘ Nurses have a key role in screening, managing and supporting dysphagic patients.

References

Aviv JE, Martin JH, Jones ME (1994) Age-related changes in pharyngeal and supraglottic sensation. *Ann Otol Rhinol Laryngol* **103**: 749–52

Aviv JE (2000) Prospective randomized outcome study of endoscopy versus modified barium swallow in patients with dysphagia. *Laryngoscope* **110**(4): 563–74

Aviv JE, Kaplan ST, Thomson JE *et al* (2000) The safety of flexible endoscopic evaluation of swallowing with sensory testing (FEESST): an analysis of 500 consecutive evaluations. *Dysphagia* **15**(1): 39–44

Axelsson K, Norberg A, Asplund K (1984) Eating after a stroke — towards an integrated view. *Int J Nurs Stud* **21**(2): 93–9

Bastian RW (1991) Videoendoscopic evaluation of patients with dysphagia: an adjunct to the modified barium swallow. *Otolaryngol Head Neck Surg* **104**: 339–50

Bath PMW, Bath FJ, Smithard DG (2000) *Interventions for dysphagia in acute stroke*. (Cochrane Review). In: The Cochrane Library 2. Update software, Oxford

Bleach NR (1993) The gag reflex and aspiration: a retrospective analysis of 120 patients assessed by videofluoroscopy. *Clin Otolaryngol* **18**: 303–7

British Medical Association (1999) *Withholding and Withdrawing Life-Prolonging Medical Treatment. Guidance for Decision-making*. BMJ Publishing, London

British Society of Gastroenterology (1996) *Guidelines on Artificial Nutrition Support*. British Society of Gastroenterology, London

Carr EK, Hawthorn PJ (1988a) Lip function and eating after a stroke: a nursing perspective. *J Adv Nurs* **13**: 447–51

Carr EK, Hawthorn PJ (1988b) Observation of eating skills after a stroke: dribbling food and chewing. *Clin Rehabil* **2**: 183–9

Chaudhuri G, Hildner C, Brady S, Hutchins E, Abadilla E, Aliga N (2000) Cardiovascular effects of the supraglottic swallowing procedure in stroke patients with dysphagia. *Dysphagia* **15**: 106

Celifarco A, Gerard G, Faegenburg D, Burakoff R (1990) Dysphagia as the sole manifestation of bilateral strokes. *Am J Gastroenterol* **8**: 610–30

Daniels SK, Brailey K, Foundas AL (1999) Lingual discoordination and dysphagia following acute stroke: analysis of lesion location. *Dysphagia* **14**: 85–92

Daniels SK, Brailey K, Priestly DH *et al* (1998) Aspiration in patients with acute stroke. *Arch Phys Med Rehabil* **79**: 14–19

Daniels SK, McAdam CP, Brailey K, Foundas AL (1997) Clinical assessment of swallowing and prediction of dysphagia severity. *Am J Speech Language Pathologists* **6**: 17–24

Davies S, Fall S, Barer D (1998) Dysphagia and nutrition after stroke: should more patients be considered for early PEG feeding? *Clin Rehabil* **12**(2): 162

Davies S, Taylor H, MacDonald A, Barer D (2001) An inter-disciplinary approach to swallowing problems in acute stroke. *Int J Communication Disorders* **36**(suppl): 357–62

Feinberg MJ (1996) A perspective on age-related changes of the swallowing mechanism and their clinical significance. *Dysphagia* **11**: 185–6

Finucane TE, Bynum JPW (1996) Use of tube feeding to prevent aspiration pneumonia. *Lancet* **348**: 1421–4

Freed ML, Freed L, Chatburn RL, Christian M (2001) Electrical stimulation for swallowing disorders caused by stroke. *Res Care* **46**(5): 466–74

Groher M (1997) *Dysphagia: Diagnosis and Management*. 3rd edn. Butterworth-Heinemann, Boston

Hargrove R (1980) Feeding the severely dysphagic patient. *J Neurosurg Nurs* **12**(2): 102–7

Hinds NP, Wiles CM (1998) Assessment of swallowing and referral to speech and language therapists in acute stroke. *Q J Med* **91**(12): 829–35

Hotaling DL (1990) Adapting the mealtime environment: setting the stage for eating. *Dysphagia* **5**: 77–83

Hudson HM, Daubert CR, Mills RH (2000) The interdependency of protein-energy malnutrition, ageing, and dysphagia. *Dysphagia* **15**(1): 31–8

Intercollegiate Working Party for Stroke for the Royal College of Physicians of London (2000) *The National Clinical Guidelines for Stroke*. RCP, London
http://www.rcplondon.ac.uk/pubs/books/ stroke/index.htm (accessed: 12 April 2001)

Kahrilas PJ, Logemann JA, Drugler C, Flanagan E (1991) Volitional augmentation of upper oesophageal sphincter opening during swallowing. *Am J Physiol* **260**: 6450–6

Kayser-Jones J, Pengilly K (1999) Dysphagia amongst nursing home residents. *Geriatr Nurs* **20**(2): 77–84

Kayser-Jones J, Schell E (1997) The effect of staffing on the quality of care at mealtime. *Nurs Outlook* **45**(2): 64–72

Kuhlemeier KV (1994) Epidemiology and dysphagia. *Dysphagia* **9**: 209

Kuhlemeier KV Yates P, Palmer JB (1998) Intra- and interrater variation in the evaluation of videofluorographic swallowing studies. *Dysphagia* **13**: 142–7

Kuhlemeier KV, Palmer JB, Rosenberg D (2001) Effect of liquid bolus consistency and delivery method on aspiration and pharyngeal retention in dysphagia patients. *Dysphagia* **16**(2): 119–22

Landis RJ, Koch GG (1977) The measurement of observer agreement for categorical data. *Biometrics* **33**: 159–74

Layne KA (1990) Feeding strategies for the dysphagic patient: a nursing perspective. *Dysphagia* **5**: 84–8

Lazzara G, Lazarus C, Logemann J (1986) Impact of thermal stimulation on the triggering of the swallow reflex. *Dysphagia* **1**: 73–7

Leder SB (1996) Gag reflex and dysphagia. *Head Neck* **18**: 138–41

Lennard-Jones JE (1998) *Ethical and Legal Aspects of Clinical Hydration and Nutritional Support*. The British Association for Parenteral and Enteral Nutrition, Maidenhead

Lim S, Lieu PK, Phua SY, Seshadri R, Venketasubramanian N, Lee SH, Choo PWJ (2001) Accuracy of bedside clinical methods compared with FEES in determining the risk of aspiration in acute stroke patients. *Dysphagia* **16**: 1–6

Lindgren S, Janzon L (1991) Prevalence of swallowing complaints and clinical findings among 50- to 79-year-old men and women in an urban population. *Dysphagia* **6**(4): 187–92

Logemann J (1998) *Evaluation and Treatment of Swallowing Disorders*. 2nd edn. Pro-Ed, Austin, Texas

Logemann JA, Kahrilas PJ, Kobara M, Vakil NB (1989) The benefit of head rotation on pharyngeal-oesophageal dysphagia. *Arch Phys Med Rehabil* **70**(10): 767–71

Logemann JA, Pauloski BR, Colangelo L, Lazarus C, Fujiu M, Kahrilas PJ (1995) Effects of a sour bolus on oropharyngeal swallowing measures in patients with neurogenic dysphagia. *J Speech Hearing Res* **38**(3): 556–63

Low J, Wyles C, Wilkinson T, Sainsbury R, (2001) The effect of compliance on clinical outcomes for patients with dysphagia on videofluoroscopy. *Dysphagia* **16**(2): 123–7

Martin-Harris B, Logemann J, McMahon S, Schleicher M, Sandridge J (2000) Clinical utility of the modified barium swallow. *Dysphagia* **15**: 136–41

McLaren S (1997) Eating disabilities following stroke. *Br J Community Health Nurs* **2**(1): 9–18

Mennell S, Murcott A, Otterloo AH (1992) *The Sociology of Food, Eating, Diet and Culture*. Sage Publications, London

Neumann MJ, Meyer CT, Dutton JL, Smith R (1995) Hold that X-ray: aspirate pH and auscultation prove enteral tube placement. *J Clin Gastroenterol* **20**(4): 293–5

Nilsson H, Ekberg O, Olsson R, Hindfelt B (1998) Dysphagia in stroke: a prospective study of quantitative aspects of swallowing in dysphagic patients. *Dysphagia* **13**: 32–8

Norton B, Homer-Ward M, Donnelly MT, Long RG, Holmes GK (1996) A randomized prospective comparison of percutaneous endoscopic gastrostomy and nasogastric tube feeding after acute dysphagic stroke. *Br Med J* **312**: 13–16

Odderson IR, Keaton JC, McKenna BS (1995) Swallow management in patients on an acute stroke pathway: quality is cost-effective. *Arch Phys Med Rehabil* **76**: 1130–3

Park C, O'Neill PA, Martin DF (1997) A pilot exploratory study of oral electrical stimulation on swallow function following stroke: an innovative technique. *Dysphagia* **12**: 161–6

Park RHR, Allison MC, Lang J *et al* (1992) Randomized comparison of percutaneous endoscopic gastrostomy and nasogastric tube feeding in patients with persisting neurological dysphagia. *Br Med J* **304**: 1406–9

Payne-James JJ, Khawaja HT (1993) First choice for total parenteral nutrition: the peripheral route. *J Parenteral Enteral Nutrition* **17**(5): 467–78

Penman JP, Thomson M (1998) A review of the textured diets developed for the management of dysphagia. *J Hum Nutrition Diet* **11**: 51–60

Perez I, Smithard DG, Davies H, Kalra L (1998) Pharmacological treatment of dysphagia in stroke. *Dysphagia* **13**: 12–6

Perie S, Laccourreye L, Flahaut A *et al* (1998) Role of videoendoscopy in assessment of pharyngeal function in oropharyngeal dysphagia: comparison with videofluoroscopy and manometry. *Laryngoscope* **108**: 1712–6

Perry L, Love CP (2001) Screening for dysphagia and aspiration in acute stroke: a systematic review. *Dysphagia* **16**: 1–12

Perry L, McLaren S (2000a) Dysphagia screening, assessment and outcomes in stroke patients: phase one of an 'evidence-based practice' project. *J Clin Excellence* **1**: 201–8

Perry L, McLaren S (2000b) An evaluation of implementation of evidence-based guidelines for dysphagia screening and assessment following acute stroke: phase 2 of an evidence-based practice project. *J Clin Excellence* **2**: 147–56

Rehman HU, Knox J (2000) There is a need for regular review of swallowing ability in patients after PEG insertion to identify patients with delayed recovery of swallowing. *Dysphagia* **15**: 48

Rickman J (1998) Percutaneous endoscopic gastrostomy: psychological effects. *Br J Nurs* **7**(12): 723–9

Robbins JA, Hamilton JW, Lof GL, Kempster G (1992) Oropharyngeal swallowing in normal adults of different ages. *Gastroenterol* **103**: 823–9

Robbins JA, Levine RL, Maser A *et al* (1993) Swallowing after unilateral stroke of the cerebral cortex. *Arch Phys Med Rehabil* **74**: 1295–300

Rollins H (1997) A nose for trouble. *Nurs Times* **93**(49): 66–7

Rosenbek JC (1995) Efficacy in dysphagia. *Dysphagia* **10**: 263–7

Royal College of Speech and Language Therapists (1998) *Clinical Guidelines by Consensus for Speech and Language Therapists*. RCSLT, London

Shanahan TK, Logemann JA, Rademaker AW, Pauloski BR, Kahrilas PJ (1993) Chin-down posture effect on aspiration in dysphagic patients. *Arch Phys Med Rehabil* **74**: 736–9

Sidenvall B, Ek AC (1993) Long-term care patients and their dietary intake related to eating ability and nutritional needs: nursing staff interventions. *J Adv Nurs* **18**: 565–73

Smith HA, Lee SH, O'Neill PA, Connolly MJ (2000) The combination of bedside swallowing assessment and oxygen saturation monitoring of swallowing in acute stroke: a safe and humane screening tool. *Age Ageing* **29**: 495–9

Smithard DG, O'Neill PA, England R *et al* (1997) The natural history of dysphagia following a stroke. *Dysphagia* **12**: 188–93

Smithard DG, O'Neill PA, Park C *et al* (1998) Can bedside assessment reliably exclude aspiration following acute stroke? *Age Ageing* **27**: 99–106

Sorin R, Somers S, Austin W, Bester S (1988) The influence of videofluoroscopy on the management of the dysphagic patient. *Dysphagia* **2**: 127–35

Stratton RJ, Wright L, Frost GS (1998) Energy intakes fail to meet requirements on texture modified diets. *Proceedings of the Nutrition Society* **57**: 117A

Stroud A (1997) To evaluate the reliability of auscultation for the detection of aspiration. *Dysphagia* **12**: 118

United Kingdom Central Council for Nursing, Midwifery and Health Visiting (1997) *Responsibility for the Feeding of Patients (Registrar's letter)*. UKCC, London

Van Ort S, Phillips LR (1995) Nursing interventions to promote functional feeding. *J Gerontol Nurs* **21**(10): 6–14

Wykes R (1997) The nutritional and nursing benefits of social mealtimes. *Nurs Times* **93**(4): 32–4

Zorowitz RD, Robinson EM (1999) Pathophysiology of dysphagia and aspiration. *Top Stroke Rehabil* **6**(3): 1–16

Glossary and photographs of common oral health conditions and terminology

Richard White and Dr JM Watkins

Disorders of the oropharynx are generally exclusive in terms of appearance and nomenclature. Some, such as lichen planus, thrush and pemphigus appear elsewhere on the body and are familiar to dermatologists and genito-urinary physicians. In addition, relatively new clinical phenomena such as HIV disease and chemotherapy have oral manifestations important to both patient and carer. Successful management will involve not only an awareness of such presentations but also the need for ongoing assessment. Infectious diseases of the mouth are common, they involve a variety of organisms such as bacteria and yeasts, all of which will respond to appropriate treatment.

This chapter is intended as a brief introduction to the terminology and presentations of oral health and disease. For a more comprehensive coverage the reader is advised to consult more authoritative texts (see 'References').

Photographs reproduced by kind permission of
Dr JM Watkins MB, MS, MRCGP

Angular cheilitis: sore, raw and fissured angles of the mouth; caused by candida. Check for ill-fitting dentures. See *Figure Glossary.1.*

Aphthous ulcer: a small, superficial often painful ulcer of the mouth or pharynx; characteristically multiple and recurrent. Often associated with HIV disease. See *Figure Glossary.2.*

Candidiasis: a white, creamy area of oral mucosa and/or tongue that can easily be removed by rubbing to leave a red, raw base. Frequently seen in immunosuppressed patients and those receiving antibiotic therapy. See *Glossary Figure. 3.*

Denture stomatitis: ulceration and/or infection of the mouth attributable to dentures, whether ill fitting or unhygienic.

Dysphagia: difficulty in swallowing, sensation of food sticking in the oesophagus. Note: the assessment of the swallowing reflex is the responsibility of the physician.

Epulis: (pl. epulides) a lump on the gum due to irritation or inflammation of the gingival margin.

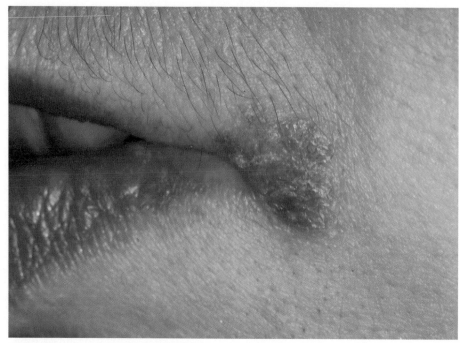

Figure Glossary.1: Angular cheilitis

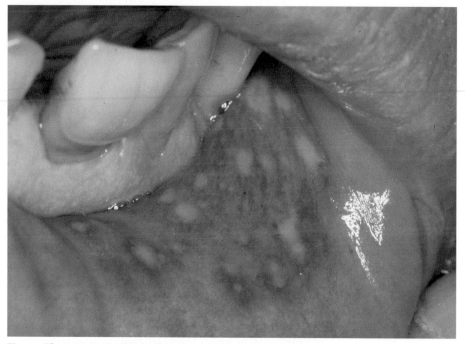

Figure Glossary.2: Apthous ulcer

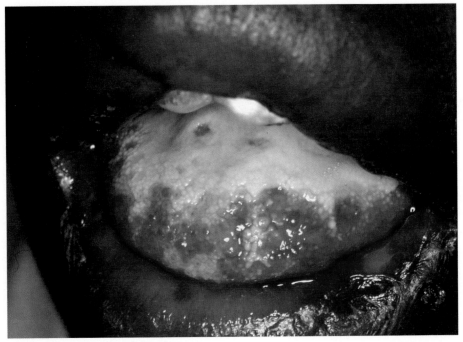

Figure Glossary.3: Candidiasis

Erythema multiforme: most usually a skin condition; rarely affects the mouth as painful erosions of the gums and palate. The Stevens-Johnson syndrome qv is a variant. Attributed to an infection or an adverse drug response.

Gingivitis: any inflammatory condition of the gingivae. There are numerous forms, subject to expert assessment. See *Figure Glossary.4.*

Glossitis: inflammation of the tongue with loss of the characteristic surface papillae, a red, smooth-surfaced tongue. Associated with nutritional deficiencies, dehydration, drug side-effect.

Glossodynia: burning pain in the tongue, associated with diabetes, smoking, xerostomia, clinical depression, drug side-effects.

Halitosis: bad breath; due to infection of the oral cavity (gingivitis) or respiratory tract, liver or kidney disease. Halitosis can occur in the mouth, nasopharynx, lungs, and gastrointestinal tract.

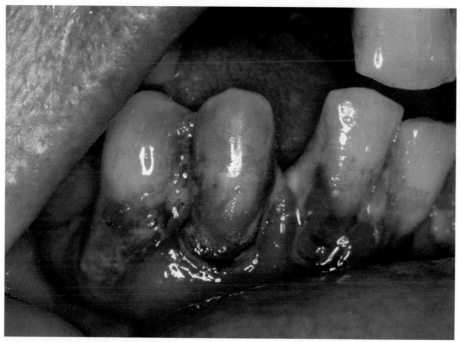

Figure Glossary.4: Gingivitis

Herpes labialis: an acute vesicular eruption of Herpes simplex on the lips. Exacerbated during febrile illnesses such as pneumonia.

Leucoplakia: any white mucosal lesion that cannot be easily removed by rubbing. If the area has a red (erythematous) component it is erythroplakia, a pre-malignant condition.

Lichen planus: a relatively common benign disease of the skin and mucous membranes, occurs mainly in females in the age range of thirty to eighty. It is an inflammatory pruritic disease with characteristic violaceous lesions with fine white streaks. It can be erosive involving the tongue and/or mucous membranes. See *Figure Glossary.4.*

Macroglossia: abnormal enlargement of the tongue, indicative of systemic diseases such as myxoedema and amyloidosis.

Pemphigus/ pemphigoid: are known as 'bullous' or blistering diseases. Lesions are blisters to both the mouth and the skin; these can burst to leave erosions.

Periodontitis: inflammation of the periodontium.

Perleche: angular cheilitis.

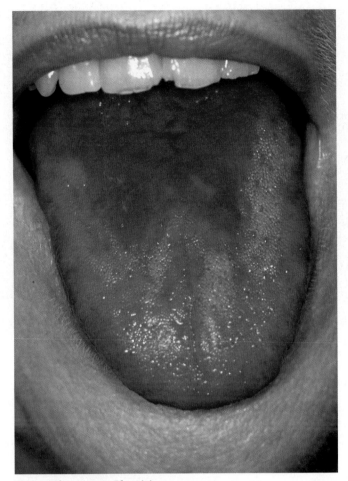

Figure Glossary.5: Glossitis

Polyp: scar tissue often produced in response to trauma (also look for bruising, tooth loss, etc.).

Stevens-Johnson syndrome: a serious form of stomatitis seen as severe blistering of the lips, of unknown aetiology, associated with drugs such as antibiotics.

Stomatitis: a wide range of conditions including ulceration and infection of the mucous membranes. Causes range from infection by bacteria (Vincent's infection), viruses (Herpes simplex) or yeast (Candida) to radio- and chemotherapies, anaemia, scurvy, immunosuppression (eg. HIV), and drug side-effects (see *Table 1.4*).

Thrush: also candidiasis.

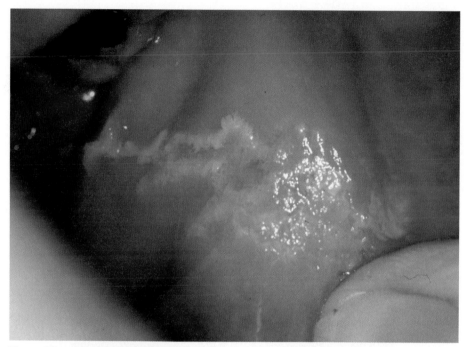

Figure Glossary.6: Lichen planus

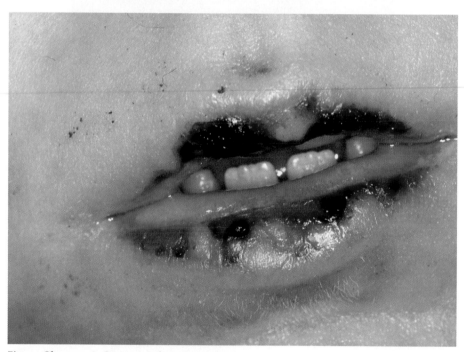

Figure Glossary.7: Stevens Johnson syndrome

Xerostomia: dry mouth, due to reduced salivary output usually through dehydration, disease (eg. Sjogren's syndrome), radiotherapy or drug side-effects (eg. some antihistamines). Can also be the result of anxiety or stress. Requires meticulous oral hygiene and appropriate treatment.

References

Edgar M, Harris M, eds (1977) *Clinical Oral Science.*Wright, London
Cohen LK, Gift HC (1995) *Disease Prevention and Oral Health Promotion.* Blackwell, Munksgaard
Faller RV, Karger (2000) *Assessment of Oral Health.* S Karger, Basel
Scully C (2000) *ABC of Oral Health.* BMJ Books, London

Table Glossary. I: Assessment of common oral conditions for nurse prescribers (Preparations and drugs in bold are those currently prescribable by qualified nurse prescribers)

Conditions	Assessment			Action		
	Common symptoms	Visual examination	Other information	Advice and treatment	Referral	Follow-up
Teething	Possibly distress Mild pyrexia Excess saliva Tendency to chew on objects No other illness	Slight redness of gums, evidence of tooth erupting	Baby teeth generally appear 6–30 months And adult teeth from 5–6 years	**Paracetamol oral suspension** for 24 hours **Lignocaine-based teething gels** Keep mouth clean	If persists see GP in case other cause of ill health	Ensure symptoms resolve Time for oral hygiene instruction: brush with thin smear of fluoride paste
Dental pain due to toothache or dental abscess	Sensitive to hot and cold stimuli Constant throbbing pain	May be evidence of tooth decay but a filling may obscure any evidence of decay	Dental history	Urgent dental attendance Suitable **analgesia**, eg. **paracetamol** or **aspirin** if delay in dental appointment	General dental practitioner or local emergency dental service or use NHS direct	Encourage dental attendance to com- plete care Supportive dietary and hygiene advice Use fluoride tooth- paste
Gum infection	Bad taste in mouth Dull pain Swollen gums Bleeding on brushing	Red and swollen gums: widespread or localised	Tooth cleaning history— people often stop cleaning when gums are bleeding or painful	Good oral hygiene Limited use of **analgesics** if required as interim measure Chlorhexidine (Corsodyl) mouthwash	Seek dental care including professional cleaning and oral hygiene instruction	Support oral health care regimen advised — note behaviour change is not easy
Dry mouth	Often associated with radiotherapy to head and neck, salivary gland disease or drug interactions Difficulty in eating biscuits Takes constant sips of water	Reduced saliva Sticky or frothy saliva Lack of pooling of saliva in the floor of the mouth	Check if patient is sucking sugary sweets — these will lead rapidly to tooth decay if the client has natural teeth. Check patient's medication	Determine if cause can be eliminated Consider prescribing **Thymol/Glycerin** mouthwash (interim). Ensure that patient receives regular dental care	Liaise with GP if due to medication Liaise with GP or GDP for referral to specialist if persistent under- lying cause	If have natural teeth, clients need support to prevent tooth decay — avoidance of frequent sugary intake, good oral hygiene, saliva sub- stitutes etc including plain water

Table Glossary.1: cont.

Mouth ulcers	Painful ulcer or painless ulcer	Check if single or multiple, recurrent or first such episode. Is it associated with edge of a denture or sharp tooth? Risk factors for oral cancer include tobacco and alcohol (especially together)	Beware of a painless ulcer or an ulcer which persists for more than 3 weeks as this may be evidence of malignancy. If there is general malaise then the ulcers may be viral. If recurrent then apthous stomatitis	Leave dentures out as much as possible. Advise on use of OTC medications, eg. **corsodyl mouth-wash or orabase ointment**. Limited use of **analgesics**, eg. paracetamol, particularly if viral infection	Assist with dental appointment, particularly if there are concerns about possible malignancy	Ensure that the mouth ulcer has resolved completely and under-lying condition (eg. denture) has been dealt with
Candida (thrush) in baby	Mother experiencing pain on breastfeeding	Baby has typical oral candida lesions		**Nystatin oral suspension**		Support mother to continue breast-feeding
Candida (thrush) in child or adult	Pain under top denture or painful soft tissues in immunocompromised patient. Extensive white patches	Red patch under denture or white patch on soft tissues which, when rubbed off, leaves red bleeding	May be associated with recent antibiotic or found in an already immunocompromised patient, eg. post radio-therapy or use of inhalers	Good denture hygiene (if appropriate) Consider **Nystatin pastilles** if no other underlying concerns or treatment approved by specialist Wash out mouth after inhalers (if used)	Liaison with GP or GDP especially if underlying condition to ensure that you support appropriate care for this client and they seek specialist advice if necessary Check diabetes if no other known cause	Support good oral hygiene and dental care Support client in dealing with under-lying condition
Cracked lips	Painful cracked lips	Possibly fissured	If denture-wearer, may need new dentures	**Paraffin wax** Miconazole gel to lips and mouth	Seek dental check-up if persists	Support dental attendance if required
Bad breath	Patient or others complain of bad breath	May be evidence of poor oral hygiene and debris	Usually poor oral hygiene and infection in mouth	Improve oral hygiene Chlorhexidine (Corsodyl) mouth-wash	Seek dental check-up if it does not resolve	Support good oral hygiene and dental care
Furred tongue	Furred, hairy or coated tongue	Thick coating on tongue which may even be black and 'hairy'	Poor oral hygiene Smoking	Clean tongue with toothbrush or scraper Reduce smoking	Seek dental check-up if it does not resolve	Support good oral hygiene

Reproduced by kind permission of Jenny Gallagher and Jean Rowe

Index